A Gateway to Daily Life Yoga

Masahiro Oki

Okido Natural Health Education Trust CIO

Originally published in Japanese with the title '*Seikatsu Yoga Nyūmon, shinshin ga umare kawaru hon*' by Tokuma Shoten Publishing Co. in 1979. Copyright © 1979 Masahiro Oki

This translation is permitted by the copyright owner of the original book.

First published in the United Kingdom in 2024 by
Okido Natural Health Education Trust CIO
www.okidoyoga.org.uk

Copyright © 2024 Tomoko Mori

A CIP catalogue record for this book is available from the British Library.

ISBN: 978-1-0687783-0-8

Printed and bound in the United Kingdom

Translation: Tomoko Mori
Translation assistance: Junko Furugori and Hiroyuki Mori
Photography: Hiroyuki Mori
Modelling and proofreading: dedicated contributors

This book is not intended to provide a substitute to professional medical advice. Any use of the information and exercises herein is at the reader's discretion and risk. The copyright owner, translator and publisher disclaim any liability directly or indirectly from the use of the contents in this book.

Contents

I Daily Life Yoga Transforms You
— Philosophy of yoga discipline

II How to Control Our Mind and Body through Yoga
— A key to good use and care of the mind and body

III Yoga during Your Commute
— How to enjoy a crowded train

IV Yoga in the Office
— To have good relationships and improve work efficiency

V Yoga in Your Home
— Make your home a yoga *dōjō*

VI Meditation Discipline Leads You to the State of *Mu*
—How to deepen and expand the self

About the author

Japanese yoga master, Masahiro Oki, was born in 1919 (officially registered as 1921). Not born robust, he suffered from various illnesses for many years. Through his parents and their connections, he was brought up in an atmosphere of spiritual discipline. When he was about 12 years old, he first heard the term 'yoga' from Sayadaw U Ottama, a great monk and the father of Burmese independence, and learnt that yoga was the path Shakyamuni had followed.

In his youth, following his father's death, he became a special agent for the Japanese government, underwent various special training and went to Mongolia, China, India and Arabia. Through his work, he experienced religious training in Lamaism, Taoism, Islam, Buddhism, Judaism and Christian temples, and learnt Eastern and Western medicine as well as ancient Indian and Arabian medical methods. In India, he stayed at Mahatma Gandhi's ashram for some time, where the Mahatma told him, "Shakyamuni, Christ and other saints became enlightened by practising yoga. I practise it, too. Studying yoga and religion is not about reading books, but about putting the teachings into practice." By observing and imitating the Mahatma's lifestyle, Oki came to understand that yoga is about living in a balanced way.

After World War Ⅱ, he aspired to become a peacemaker and lived a life of disciplining himself in devoted service and humbleness, based in Japan's Hokuriku region. In 1951, he went to India as Japan's representative to UNESCO's international service mission for peacebuilding, where he served others in the medical and welfare fields. While living such a life, he realised that the more he tried to devote himself to service the more he became aware of the ugliness, lowliness and weakness of his mind, and so came to seek how he could live a life of holiness like

Shakyamuni and Mahatma Gandhi. He was deeply moved that the teachings of yoga had led Shakyamuni and Mahatma Gandhi to enlightenment. During this period, he discovered that he had intestinal cancer and began to practise yoga in earnest with the aim of transforming his mind and body.

He returned to Japan in 1955. He ran yoga activities throughout Japan to spread the spirit of gratitude and service. In addition, from 1960 onwards, he was often invited to lecture on Eastern philosophy and medicine in various countries of the West.

He named the yoga he studied as 'Yoga for the Search of Truth' and established Oki Yoga Shūdōjō in Mishima in 1967. From this base, he spread Oki Yoga (or Oki-dō Yoga, or Okido Yoga) both nationally and internationally, and guided many people.

Oki Yoga is a modern and comprehensive interpretation of yoga that links many areas of human life. It teaches utilising all aspects of life as methods for training body, mind and spirit, and aims to search for truth about how humans should live.

On 25 July 1985, the day after the European Summer Camp 1985 was completed, Masahiro Oki died in the Adriatic Sea, in Italy.

Note:
This page is not part of the translation of the original Japanese book. The translator wrote it referring to the following sources:
  Common statements in the author introductions of various books written by Masahiro Oki in Japanese, as well as his own accounts within them, including: 'Jissen Meisō Yoga (実践冥想ヨガ [†]Practical Meditation Yoga)' published by Nichibō Shuppansha, 1978; 'Ikite-iru Shūkyō-no Hakken (生きている宗教の発見 [†]Discovery of A Living Religion)' published by Takei Shuppan, 1985
          [†]: The English titles are just given for the reader, but not official ones.
  An article on the Masahiro Oki Memorial Museum website,
  https://okimasahiro.yoga/index.php/history/   Accessed on 5 August 2024

Other references:
  'Meditation Yoga' published by Japan Publication INC, 1978
  'Meditation Yoga' published by Stichting Okido Yoga Dojo Nederland, 2001

Translator's foreword

In 1977 in Japan, when I was a university student, I read one of Masahiro Oki's books for the first time. Impressed by the comprehensive content, I went to his yoga *dōjō* in Mishima during that winter holiday. In April 1980, a year after graduating, I started to learn Okido Yoga as a resident student under him. I listened to many of his lectures on what yoga is and what it aims for. I learnt that yoga is not exercise manuals or treatment methods but a synthesis of philosophy and practical methods, and that this message of Master Oki was Okido Yoga.

The master appointed me to work for a charity promoting Okido Yoga in England that was newly being established, and so I came over to England in 1984.

I felt unequal to the task of representing the holistic synthesis of Okido Yoga. However, I worked my best for the charity as an Okido Yoga teacher, with the master's words: 'Make a sincere group however small it is'. Countless events and encounters, problems and achievements, have occurred during these 40 years. One of the achievements has been to nurture trustful human relationships among people who participated in Okido Yoga activities to do something good for themselves and others. For me, Okido Yoga philosophy sounded full of abstract ideas 40 years ago. But it is now becoming grounded life wisdom while I have been subconsciously applying it all these years in daily life, especially in life's most difficult situations. Now I see that every word expressed in Okido Yoga philosophy contains many layers of deep meaning, which gradually reveal themselves as life is lived sincerely.

The master encouraged us to study and practise yoga as a whole, while gaining many direct experiences in life, and to develop our own individuality as well as harmonious cooperation with others.

Masahiro Oki's Japanese book '*Seikatsu Yoga Nyūmon - shinshin ga umare kawaru hon* (生活ヨガ入門 – 心身が生まれ変わる本)' explains his philosophy of yoga from profound as well as practical perspectives, which we can utilise in our daily life. I am glad that the English translation is now completed with the title 'A Gateway to Daily Life Yoga', being published in the 40th anniversary year of the charity. My English language is not good enough to do this thorough work, and so two native English language users, Junko Furugori and Hiroyuki Mori, assisted my work, devoting enormous time and energy. Also, I would like to acknowledge Mizue Tamaki, who had sat by the master's side and translated his lectures for many years, and, since then, continued to explore suitable ways to explain in English the specific terms used in Okido Yoga philosophy. This helped my work greatly. Many other people supported me in various ways to publish this book, as well as to work a part of the charity for these past 40 years. My sincere gratitude goes to all these people.

Lastly, I would like to mention the following: Many exercises are introduced in this book, which are loyally translated from the original Japanese text. At fundamental points throughout the book, Masahiro Oki repeats that every person is different and each person should apply stimulations suitable for themselves. For me, I consider the introduced exercises as examples, focus on the meaning of each one, and adjust to a degree or devise another way in order to bring me a suitable stimulation. I apply the same adjustable way for the mental aspects mentioned in the book.

I hope this translation will be useful for many people.

August 2024   Tomoko Mori

Explanatory notes

Specific Words
When the following words appear in this book, an asterisk * is placed in front of each word. Please find their meanings here.

Reference: **'Meditation Yoga'**, the English translation of Masahiro Oki's Japanese book '冥想ヨガ入門', translated by Mizue Tamaki and Belia Biesheuvel, published by Stichting Okido Yoga Dojo Nederland, 2001.

busshō
(Japanese, 仏性) The following is from the book 'Meditation Yoga': "The literal translation of *busshō* is 'buddha nature'. According to Masahiro Oki, it means the 'original human desire for correctness'. He explained that this desire is latent within all of us, and we must reawaken and cultivate this desire through effort. Masahiro Oki says that *busshō* is something that is specific to human beings."

discipline
In this book, this word does not mean 'to train somebody to obey rules or a code of behaviour enforced by punishment'. It means 'to train oneself in self-motivated practice for personal development. It is particularly used to translate *gyōhō* (行法). *Gyōhō* is a Japanese word that originally means 'to practise Buddhism', especially, regarding esoteric Buddhism. Okido Yoga is not a sect of Buddhism, but a synthesis founded on many great teachings and experiences that Masahiro Oki learnt worldwide. Okido Yoga is independent from any established religion. However, based on the Japanese background, he used the word '*gyōhō*' to refer to the activities he adopted in his yoga *dōjō*. Therefore, in Okido Yoga '*gyōhō*' means 'a practical discipline of searching for

truth'. This meaning is applied to terms such as yoga discipline, Meditation discipline, and so on.

dōjō

(Japanese, 道場) This word consists of two characters: *dō* (道 the way) and *jō* (場 a place). The following text is from the book 'Meditation Yoga': "A *dōjō* is a residential training centre where physical training and mental training are integrated into daily life, whether it be a centre for learning the tea ceremony, cooking, martial arts, music or painting. These arts have the purpose of improving a person and helping them to find truth—through communal life with the master and senior trainees."

kansha, zange, geza, hōshi, aigyō

(Japanese, 感謝, 懺悔, 下座, 捧仕, 愛行) These Japanese words respectively mean 'unconditional gratitude', 'self-reflective repentance', 'humbleness with respect', 'devoted service' and 'practising love'. Masahiro Oki uses these five words as a set when he talks about the attitude of mind-heart for humans to develop their personality.

Meditation

(Japanese, 冥想) The following is from the book 'Meditation Yoga': "The Japanese word *meisō* is usually used to mean sitting meditation. When he uses this word, Masahiro Oki is referring to the holistic yoga of ten steps integrated into daily life. In the original Japanese version of this book [note: the book 'Meditation Yoga'], he uses a different Japanese character *mei* to the usual character used for this word. He uses the character 冥, though 瞑 is usually used. The character Masahiro Oki uses can be literally translated as 'dark', 'invisible' or 'deep'. In Masahiro Oki's definition of *meisō* it contains the meaning to 'see widely and

deeply', and this includes that which cannot be seen: to 'see, sense or feel the invisible'. When the word 'meditation' appears beginning with a small 'm', this means sitting meditation. (This is not meant to imply that sitting meditation does not also strive towards deeper revelation.) For the sake of clarity, when the word 'Meditation' appears beginning with a capital 'M', this is used to mean Masahiro Oki's definition."
The same is applied in 'A Gateway to Daily Life Yoga'.

mikkyō, kengyō (or kenkyō)
(Japanese, 密教, 顕教) Literally translated, mikkyō is esoteric teaching, whereas kengyō is exoteric teaching. Regarding Masahiro Oki's definition, the following text is from the book 'Meditation Yoga': "There are two types of teaching, kengyō and mikkyō. Yoga still keeps to the mikkyō tradition, while other teachings have become kengyō. Kengyō means a teaching or religion in which a text is adhered to. In mikkyō there is no text. You use yourself as the text, and you learn through experience, through facts. Following the mikkyō path means that you are your own teacher and are not dependent on anyone. You do not depend on, nor believe, theories, doctrines, 'common sense' or custom."

mind-heart
The Japanese word 'kokoro (心)' means the integration of intellect, heart, emotion, spirit, consciousness and the subconscious, that is to say, both the source of these functions and the functions themselves. Depending on the context, it can be translated into different English words such as heart, mind, mentality, emotion, feeling and spirit. Each of these English words also has a specific Japanese expression other than kokoro. However, normally, it is not necessary to distinguish between them. Traditionally, in Okido

Yoga, the word 'mind-heart' is adopted as a translation of *kokoro*. The same is applied in 'A Gateway to Daily Life Yoga'.

mu

(Japanese, 無) The literal translation is nothingness. According to Masahiro Oki's explanation, the state of 'mu' is not 'nothingness', but it means that all exists in complete harmony, which therefore feels as if nothing exists.

the *mu*-mind, *mushin*

(Japanese, 無心) This means 'the mind of non-attachment to pre-conceived judgement'.

religion, religious

Masahiro Oki expresses his philosophy saying that the purpose and value of religion is beyond the name or form of any system, and he uses the word 'religion' to refer to 'what teaches the most fundamentally important thing in life'. By the word 'religious', Masahiro Oki does not mean 'relating to an established religion or believing in it'. He means 'with a spirit similar in quality to that of religion beyond name and form'.

With no asterisk in front, these words are used in a usual sense.

Foreign Words

Japanese and Sanskrit words sometimes appear in this book. The format used in the book 'Meditation Yoga' has been adopted for this book. Except names and generally known terms, Japanese words are written in an italic sans serif typeface (for example, *kokoro*) and Sanskrit words are written in an italic serif typeface (for example, *āsana*). To indicate the long sound, a macron is used over *o* and *u* for Japanese, and over *a*, *i*, and *u* for Sanskrit. Other diacritical marks are omitted.

Preface

To utilise yoga in daily life

I have written many books on yoga. However, all of them were focused on either the mind or body. There was no book in which I concretely explained how to utilise yoga in our daily life.

Yoga is originally a philosophy that teaches how to balance the mind, body and lifestyle following natural law, and is also a system of methods to put this philosophy into practice.

Happiness cannot be attained unless the mind, body and lifestyle are stable and balanced without forcing or wasting our energy. To do this, it is important that we give ourselves things that suit us, in ways that are suitable, and only as much as we need. If we just imitate somebody else's way or are obsessed with various theories, we will never be able to discover ourselves. We must discover ourselves and live by following natural law if we want to unite our joy with that of others.

I teach that the most natural life in accordance with the providence of the universe is a life of 'practising love', and that it is a life with 'unconditional gratitude', 'self-reflective repentance', 'humbleness with respect' and 'devoted service'. Only when we live like this can we attain true happiness.

There are various aspects in our daily life, and so, in this book, I will talk about the idea of yoga in family life and explain relationships between couples as well as between parents and children. Also, I will explain diet, recovery from tiredness, and so on.

In the aspect of work, I will explain how to view work from a yogic perspective and deal with it, and also talk about relationships at work according to different types of people.

16

Of course, I will also introduce yoga's unique practical methods regarding how to use the body and mind, which will be helpful in general life.

If we only practise the training methods of yoga *discipline without knowing its philosophy, we will unlikely receive their real effects. Therefore, I will explain yoga in 10 stages so that you will come to know yoga's *Meditation *discipline to deepen and expand your being.

It has been 42 years since I started aiming to be a true *religious person. Owing to consistent search for truth, I have come to understand that there is nothing simple in the world, and that what I thought would be solved simply cannot be easily done.

This book states that true health, beauty, enlightenment, happiness or peace will not be attained unless you adopt 'yoga' in all aspects of your lifestyle. I hope this will be of some help for you to see that yoga is not just a method for beauty or health, or a mysterious training method, but that it is a scientific and comprehensive system of philosophy and practice.

Yoga is *mikkyō, an esoteric teaching. In *mikkyō, we perceive everything as an object of learning and acquire truth through direct experience.

The content of this book is what I have come to realise based on my life experience. I will be most happy if you, the reader, can use it to attain a happy life.

November 1979 (*Shōwa* 54)   Masahiro Oki

I

Daily Life Yoga Transforms You
- Philosophy of yoga discipline

Yoga is a means of restoring humanity

Looking at trees or flowers in well-maintained parks or gardens, we cannot tell if they are happy or not, or hurt in some way.

However, when we see some greenish things covered in the exhaust fumes of passing cars and surrounded by iron guardrails, we wonder if they are fully living their lives. We cannot help but feel sorry for those dirty trees and flowers.

All living creatures are products of nature. Therefore, if they, whether plants or animals, remain wild, we as outsiders will not need to say anything. We should only be concerned about those creatures that are placed in artificial environments.

There is no doubt that human beings are also originally a product of nature. In ancient times, there would have been no special early childhood education or fiercely competitive school entrance examinations. However, even a slight wound could cause loss of life because there was no such thing as medical science. Also, humans could not fly faster than a hawk or run on the ground faster than a horse.

We humans have culture. This is a privilege only given to us. But cultural life is not a natural life. No matter how we seem to adapt to our cultural life, human beings, a product of nature, leave some non-adaptable parts behind, which may lead to irreversible problems.

Yoga is the research of how we humans, who are children of nature and basically controlled by nature, can live our cultural and civilised life.

Bizarre-looking physical training is sometimes done in yoga. However, please keep in mind that it is also a means to restore the original human nature which has become dormant and distorted in our cultural and civilised life. We can list as many harms of cultural and civilised life as we can think of.

For example, obesity. When I was a child, there was no such phrase as 'an obese child'. Obese children are now abundant everywhere. Obesity in adults can be a cause of heart disease or diabetes.

The harms of civilisation extend to non-human creatures: plants and livestock. Some livestock animals suffer from constipation, diarrhoea or liver problems as humans do. This is because they live an unnatural life, or rather, they are kept in an unnatural way. Nowadays, some dogs even seem to have neurosis.

Historically, practitioners of yoga recognised the harms of civilisation and disciplined themselves to seek salvation for humanity. It is said to date back 5,000 or 6,000 years. India has the remains of such training.

Humans cannot abandon everything and return to beings of wild nature. It was so 5,000 years ago, and it is still the same.

Therefore, yoga has been researching what the most ideal state of the human mind is, what state the body should be in, and how our lifestyle and environment should be in order to keep a state in which both ourselves and others can be happy. Yoga asks how humans should live as a civilisation.

In summary, yoga is a quest for the freedom for us to live as a civilisation.

God is within the self

The original meaning of 'yoga' is to unite or yoke. So, what does it unite? It unites you and God. It unites you and the truth. Words such as God or truth can sound difficult, but put simply, being united with God or the truth means that you have become a true being. In other words, human beings live as true human beings. One lives as oneself. Shakyamuni, meaning 'Sage of the Shakya clan', is also called Buddha. Buddha means a free person who has developed the *busshō* (仏 性). It means someone who has acquired true freedom of mind, true freedom of body, and true freedom of lifestyle.

In the quest for the development of the *busshō* and freedom in life, what should one do with one's body and mind? This is what yoga calls self-development. There is no textbook for it. There are textbooks or scripts in various other disciplines, teachings or religions, but there is nothing in yoga. Searching for true freedom, each person must experience and self-study everything. The self is the one who saves or punishes the self.

There is no such thing as heaven or hell. If anything, the self is the creator of heaven or hell. 'God is within the self' —this is the greatest characteristic of yoga.

In ancient Indian yoga, they renounced the world in search of human freedom. This was a bare lifestyle away from all attachments, in which they neither belonged to nor possessed anything. And they sought a way of true life through their intellectual and physical experience.

In modern day yoga, we do not do this. But what it has in common with ancient Indian yoga is that we seek to learn and acquire through our daily life what we humans have in common and what our personalities are.

In yoga, which has no textbook and must be self-studied, we have no choice but to learn step by step. We can start off with a familiar topic such as researching how to sit comfortably for the freedom of our body. We know that what is good for the body is also good for the mind. Anyway, we can progress based on our experience, with no rush, according to our own capacity. In yoga practices, an unbreakable rule is 'not to force, not to waste energy, and to continue learning'. Through practices, we learn what brings freedom and what is natural.

Eventually, each of us will find a suitable way of life. You will be able to cultivate and use your being as it suits you. Living by imitating someone else seems easy at first glance but it is actually hard. You will find a way that suits you, both at work and at home, and become your own master in every situation. It will also be possible to make your work your own.

You will become able to see the difference between what you need when climbing a mountain and what you need when descending a mountain. You will become able to see the difference between what nutrition to take when it is bright and what nutrition to take when it is dark. In other words, you will become able to handle daily life situations freely.

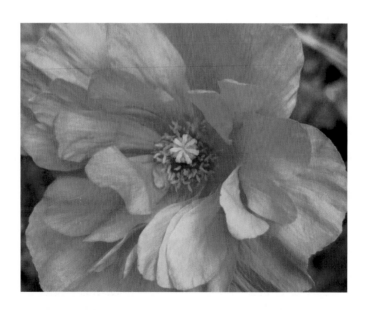

Yoga teaches: God is within the self

The three major principles of yoga are Change, Balance and Stability

As a result of pursuing how human beings, who have culture, can live freely in harmony with natural law, yoga has reached the following principles, which is common to everyone:
(1) Change
(2) Balance (Harmony)
(3) Stability
These are the three principles.

These principles mean that we are living while changing, balancing and maintaining stability. Living like this follows natural law that is common to both body and mind. If we go against it, our body becomes ill, our mind becomes troubled, and our life shows unhappiness.

In yoga, we give importance to Change. In other words, we should not have attachment to things. In the case of the body, it is in such flow that what we eat is excreted. Stagnation is not good. Habits or customs can cause stagnation.

Nature moves like the changes of the four seasons. Human customs and manners also change inexorably.

The natural and social environment constantly moves. All things are in a state of flux. It is natural that people who live in these environments also change. A beautiful youth will also have grey hair in decades. Yoga is first of all wary of losing sight of this unavoidable change and going into a stagnant, addicted or attached state.

The second principle of yoga is Balance. In other words, we should not be one-sided or partial. Work versus home, tension versus relaxation, right versus left, acid versus alkali, culture and civilisation versus nature—yoga always seeks balance. Most yoga practices are for restoring balance and correcting distortion.

Currently, because we human beings live a cultural and social life, our natural mental and physical functions are restrained and restricted. Even though humans originally have no class or discrimination, we are entangled in them. The major challenge of yoga is how to break free from that and create balance between humans as natural beings and humans as cultural beings.

Let me give a more familiar example about balance. Yoga teaches us to have 'a small meal of diverse foods' regarding diet. Yoga does not say by any means that only a vegetarian diet is the best. In my yoga *dōjō, people who are overweight by eating too much are guided to food-reducing or fasting in order to understand through experience the necessity of a small meal. This is also based on the idea of balance. In contrast to normal jogging, which is running forwards only, the jogging in my *dōjō includes running sideways, backwards, and so on. All of this comes from the principle of balance.

What does the third principle, Stability, mean? It means not being anxious or unstable. It means that you are not at a loss and that things suit you. You are stable when you live in the way that suits you.

If you are a woman and try to be like a man, you will be unstable, because it does not suit you. If you imitate one of your friends, you will be unstable. Living as a unique individual on earth brings you stability. If you act as if you know what you don't know, you will be unstable, because it betrays your true self.

It seems far from the image of the word 'stability', but I hope you can see that living as a unique individual leads to stability. Take fashion as an example. If you choose something that doesn't suit you, it will bring uneasy feelings to people around you. This shows the instability of the person wearing the outfit.

Stability means that we are aware of the lifestyle that we should adopt for ourselves and live in that way. Living a life that makes us most happy is also a form of health management. Let me explain this with a more understandable example.

Take nutrition as an example. Because individuality is the difference in temperament and constitution, the key to your nutrition is in understanding what kind of food you should eat. Eating the same food as other people does not always provide you with nutrition. Nutrition that is generally talked about is a theory and standard. Therefore, you must find what is directly connected to you.

Whether it is the way you exercise or work, you must discover how to make it your own. Anything that doesn't suit you will mean doing things forcibly or wasting energy, which causes instability.

No one should sit in the same way. You must sit in a way that suits you. I teach students who come to my *dōjō*, individually, 'You should sit in this way', 'You should breathe in this way', 'You should eat this kind of food', 'You should take this kind of mental attitude', 'You should work in this way', and so on. The teaching method of yoga is to guide students to learn and acquire what is true according to their individuality.

Yoga is happiness training

Up to this point, I have said that the purpose of yoga is to make the most of oneself and live freely and that for this purpose one must create of oneself someone who can live a life that matches natural law, based on the three principles: Change, Balance (Harmony) and Stability.

In order to live a life that meets this purpose and the three principles, we have no choice but to progress step by step. Yoga seeks neither miracles nor heavenly revelations. Yoga teaches principles and conclusions. These are: ①unifying the body (unified body); ②unifying the mind (unified mind), and ③breathing to harmonise the mind and body (harmonised breath).

When speaking of yoga, everyone most likely thinks of various poses. Some look like acrobatics and others look like the Great Buddha. They are one of the means and methods to keep our mind, body and breath in good condition. For example, yoga teaches us to correct a wrong way of sitting. It is because our lower back will be hurt if we sit in that way. Yoga teaches us to correct wrong diets. It is because we will be sick if we take such a diet. Yoga teaches us to correct wrong deeds. In yoga as well, mental cultivation begins with ethics such as not killing or not stealing. We should practise these obvious things first.

The *discipline of yoga is to reach the state of freedom by harmonising and unifying all the work of the visible body and invisible mind, and all the work of the conscious self and unconscious self.

To give a familiar example, when your mind is troubled, can you sleep soundly? If your physical condition is not well, you don't feel lively, do you? Adjusting the body by adjusting the work of the mind, adjusting the mind by adjusting the work of the body, and stabilising the body and mind in oneness—this is yoga.

Nowadays, with the development of medical science, electronics, and so on, some of what has been called the mystery of yoga practice is being unveiled. In other words, the benefits of yoga practice have begun to be proven scientifically.

For instance, *Meditation, which is the goal of yoga practice, is coming to be understood to some extent by measuring brain waves. The third type of brain wave, which is different from the brain waves during sleep or those when awake, can be measured. Of course, we cannot say that it gives a complete explanation about *Meditation, but I think it shows that yoga is not magic but very natural human training.

So far, we have been tending to take up the rudimentary and physical parts of yoga, such as yoga which improves the conditions of the stomach or intestines or yoga which helps you lose weight. This may be a good thing from one perspective because the interest in yoga grows and helps it spread. However, it is worrying from the perspective of yoga's aim, which is enlightenment. The true aim is to develop and enlighten oneself to one's best and to become someone who can give joy to others.

From the beginning, I have been consistently teaching yoga focusing on the yoga which guided Shakyamuni to enlightenment.

In one phrase, yoga is 'happiness training'. This means that true happiness is given in the state of *hōetsu*[1] (法悦).

About *hatha-yoga*, basic yoga training

The difference between yoga and other religious teachings is, put simply, that yoga focuses on practices, explains the methods from the start to the goal, and aims at enlightenment, based on the idea that God is within the self. There is no forcing or wasted energy. And so, anyone can do it as long as they have the spirit to seek the truth.

For instance, Zen asks you to just sit, without explanation. Because it is impossible from the beginning to explain with words a state that is beyond words, and because it is easy to lead to unnecessary misunderstandings, Zen begins by cutting off preconceived judgements caused by words. It may work for geniuses, but it is not a method that can be applied to everyone.

In Christianity as well, they say, 'Just believe.' Certainly, these words are right. It is because faith is the *mind-heart of believing

---

[1] This Japanese word means universal joy, or joy based on universal law. The stage of *hōetsu* is explained as the final goal of yoga in Page 180 (Chapter 6).

in something without return or expectation. The will of God is beyond human judgement, and God gives each and every one of us various sufferings in order for us to grow into a wonderful and revered person. Faith is a way of life in which one feels divine love in these sufferings, joyfully accepts them as lessons given by God, and utilises them as opportunities for evolution and sanctification.

However, to 'just believe' is something impossible unless you are a person with a very heightened *mind-heart.

The reason why yoga puts importance on an unforced natural way of life is that faith should naturally arise from the daily life that has been cultivated through *discipline and training.

I explain the path of yoga from initiation to the supreme freedom, or enlightenment, in ten stages. Even when I say 'ten stages', I do not mean there is an order in value. The order is just to make explanation easier, and these ten stages are divided according to the natural process when actually practised. Essentially, all stages combine to make this path, and if any stage is missing, it will not be yoga.

Nowadays, the 'yoga' that is taught and written about looks only at certain aspects of yoga, but this partial thing is not yoga.

The essential *discipline of yoga is *Meditation *discipline, which will be described later. However, since it is difficult to practise *Meditation *discipline from the beginning, it is necessary to explain the training of the preparatory stages. The earlier stage is *hatha-yoga*, and the later stage is *rāja-yoga*.

Yama (cautions) and *niyama* (recommendations) – the first stage

The first stage is about establishing a correct attitude of *mind-heart, the content of which is consistent with all religions. *Yama* (cautions), a main component of the first stage, means 'what one must not do', and it consists of the following five teachings:

(1) _Ahimsa_ : This is the strongest teaching among _yama_. _Ahimsa_ consists of ①No killing, ②No harming, ③No violating, ④No hurting, and ⑤No ill-treating, and teaches about making the most of all things.

(2) No lying. Seeking only the truth

(3) No stealing

(4) No evil desire : It is natural to receive only what should be given. However, in the case of human beings, we often unreasonably want things that should not be given. And that is a source of stress or worry. With evil desire, we will neither have gratitude for the things we are already given, nor feel willing to make the most of them. Moreover, we humans tend to want problems to be processed and solved in our own convenient way and want things to be given just as we wish.

    Problems will only be solved as they should be. The truth is that things can only be done how they should be. We are given when we should be given, and we lose when we should lose. We meet someone or something that we should meet, whether we like it or not, and we part with someone or something that we should part with, whether we like it or not. Therefore, unless we meet and part with an unconditional mental attitude, in *mushin (*the mu-mind), we cannot be in the state of 'leaving our fate in Nature's hands'.

(5) No possession : This is the last teaching of _yama_. 'No possession' means that we are to own only what we are allowed to own naturally. What is naturally given to us is what we can possess. We don't feel burdened with what we are given naturally.

I teach that, because unreasonable desire for ownership causes suffering, we should let go of evil desire. I myself keep this as a code of my life, which gives me a very light feeling day-to-day.

'No possession' also means we should consider that everything belongs to the public. It means, for instance: my land is not 'my' land but land belonging to society and all living creatures, and my child is not 'my' child but a child who I am entrusted to take care of by society, and so on. Only when we have this *mind-heart will we be able to have respect and love for others.

The teaching of 'no possession' tells us to abandon the desire to be happy only for ourselves and care only about ourselves. The most natural way for humankind is coexistence and co-prosperity by living in cooperation, helping and teaching each other. This 'coexistence and co-prosperity' is the true balance, that is, yoga, and only here will true world peace arise.

Next, *niyama* (recommendations) means 'what one should do'.
(1) Cleanliness of mind and body
We humans become impure when we live a life which does not suit us. For example, if you eat what doesn't suit your body, your body will make blood that does not suit itself, that is to say, unclean and impure blood for you. In order to live rightly and purely, you need to find out what it means to 'live in your own way'. We must distinguish what we understand and what we don't, and we must also say that what is right is right and what is wrong is wrong. I am determined not to tell or act with lies. Human life becomes impure by living with lies.

(2) Contentment. Knowing sufficiency
The universe always gives all living creatures only what they need. Therefore, when you get sick, you should get sick. When you are given something, you should receive it. What is given to you now

is what you need most. So, it is natural and right to think like this and utilise what you are given.

(3) *Discipline

This does not mean training that brings unreasonable suffering. It means training and discipline that we humans need in order to adapt to modern, cultural and communal life and live happily while avoiding its harms.

We must be pleased that only we humans are endowed with the ability to consciously enhance our adaptability. The higher the degree of cultural life, the more unnatural it becomes and the more we come to need training. In our cultural and over-protected life, we should naturally train ourselves more than people of old times. However, due to lack of training, the number of people with physical or mental disorders is increasing.

(4)[2] Finding God

This is a teaching to see and treat everything as God, and to find and create reverence and value in all things. For example, we normally think of our feet merely as 'our feet', but when we try to find God in our feet, a spirit like that of religion arises.

Many religious sects guide people to ask God for something, but such a way is not belief but business. What makes yoga most different from other teachings is that it teaches us to find God within the self. Only those who can find God within themselves

---

[2] It is commonly known that *niyama* consists of five components. Masahiro Oki's book 'Meditation Yoga' includes all of the five components. However, the original Japanese book from which this translation is done lists only four components. Therefore, the translator believes that one of the components must have been left out by mistake. The missing component is the fourth one: Self-study. So, the correct list of *niyama* should be (1) Cleanliness of mind and body, (2) Contentment, (3) Discipline, (4) Self-study and (5) Finding God.

can find God within others. Only then can we live a reverent life as human beings. This state is called enlightenment.

Āsana (dōzen) – the second stage

While *yama* and *niyama* teach how our *mind-heart should be, *āsana* explains the theory and method of how we can train our body's stability in order to purify and cultivate our *mind-heart.

Āsana teaches us to create the posture and movements with which our body and mind are most stable in any situation, and with which we can demonstrate our capacity. The method that is practised for this purpose in a quiet way is *zazen*[3], and the method through movements is *dōzen*[4] (*āsana*). However, the word *'dōzen'* (which is my creation) is still unfamiliar, and so I usually express *āsana* as exercises. Though, the word '*āsana*' does not imply the meaning of exercises. The true purpose of yoga *dōzen* is to cultivate a stable body and mind. It is not to lose weight, gain cosmetic benefits or address physical inactivity.

Our body must always be stable. Therefore, it is not good enough that we just stand, but we must stand in our most stable posture. It is not good enough that we just squat down, but we must squat down in a way we can maximise our body's balance. This is because the body and mind affect each other immediately.

The mind and body are essentially one. For example, if you become gloomy, your stomach will become sick. On the other hand, if your stomach is in a bad condition, you will feel down. Therefore, if your *mind-heart revives, your stomach will return

---

[3] and [4] In *zazen* (座禅) and *dōzen* (動禅), *za* (座) means sitting and *dō* (動) means moving.

to its natural state, and if your physical condition is in balance, your *mind-heart will feel better. *Āsana* explains these kinds of correlations between the mind and body in detail and teaches practical methods to apply them.

The central point of balance in all postures and movements is *tanden* (丹田). It is also called *hara* (肚). Enhancing the *tanden*'s power to maintain balance enhances the stability of the brain. For this reason, yoga's physical training directly leads to the cultivation of our *mind-heart.

Prānāyāma (how to utilise vital energy) – the third stage

Prānāyāma is a method of nourishing the mind and body from inside. *Prāna* means vital energy, which is the cosmic energy generating the life force. Breathing is the function of absorbing vital energy from the nose or skin, eating is the function of absorbing vital energy from the mouth, and being positive is the function of absorbing vital energy from the mind.

Prānāyāma teaches us to take the most nutritious things by mouth, nose and thought, and to make the best use of the vital energy taken. In addition, it explains in fine detail, 'If you apply such a method, such an effect will appear'. For example, if you want to be relaxed, open your chest, create strength in your lower abdomen and put strength in exhalation. If you want to calm your *mind-heart, breathe quietly and deeply. If you cannot make a decision, create strength in your lower back and legs and breathe strongly.

Because a particular disease manifests a particular way of breathing, it is possible for the disease to heal by changing the breathing style. This principle is applied to Oki Yoga Corrective Exercises. Breath is the language of life, and so it allows us to read someone's physical and mental state. And illness or an abnormal state of mind can be helped by breathing alone. *Prānāyāma* also details nutrition and its effects.

The first four stages are referred to as *hatha-yoga*, where *hatha* means a balance between plus and minus, or, between tension and relaxation. *Hatha-yoga* also means 'yoga for strength' because it enhances, strengthens, and puts in order the functions of the mind and body. It is namely yoga for self-development. It is important to develop and enhance one's own mental and physical strength, and then to create a system that can be used freely. This is the basis of *rāja-yoga* in the fifth stage onwards.

Rāja-yoga is yoga for self-enlightenment. Its details will be explained when I talk about *Meditation *discipline in the fifth stage onwards.

Rāja-yoga and *hatha-yoga* are essentially one. *Rāja-yoga* does not exist without *hatha-yoga*, and vice versa. '*Rāj*' means 'to rule', that is to say, 'to become one's own ruler'. And, *pratyāhāra* in the fourth stage is a *discipline of autonomy in order to be one's own master.

Pratyāhāra (discipline of autonomy) – the fourth stage

This *discipline aims to develop the ability to freely control oneself both physiologically and mentally. It means 'to be one's own master' and 'to be able to be a master wherever one is'. Simply put, it is a *discipline to make oneself someone who is not swung by external stimuli.

We can control our sensory nerves, such as to see or memorise, at our own will. We can also control our motor nerves, such as to walk or grip. However, we cannot freely move our autonomic nerves (parasympathetic nerves that work during sleep or rest and sympathetic nerves that work during activity) which control the functions of the heart, gastrointestinal tract, and so on. Yoga teaches us to take advantage of the function of the autonomic nervous system and control it with our human will.

This training means to change unconscious work to conscious work. Therefore, the point is to do things consciously.

As mentioned above, it seems easier to understand *rāja-yoga* if it is explained in the chapter on *Meditation *discipline. Here, I will only introduce the key points of the stages that make up *rāja-yoga*.

※ The fifth stage - *Dhāranā*

This is a *discipline to unite the mind and body, a method of training to gather and focus one's power on something.

※ The sixth stage - *Dhyāna*

This is the basis of Japanese Zen. It is a *discipline to create the most stable state of the mind and body.

※ The seventh stage - *Bhakti*

This is a *discipline to empty the *mind-heart by surrendering oneself to God or the truth.

※ The eighth stage - *Samādhi*

This aims at connecting oneself with others, which is also called the *discipline of *sanmai* (三昧).

※ The ninth stage - *Buddhi*

This aims at cultivating the *busshō*, which is a *discipline to have the *mind-heart sanctified[5].

---

[5] Refer to Footnote 25 in Page 179 (Chapter 6).

※ The tenth stage – *Prasāda*

This is also called the *discipline of *hōetsu* or *discipline of *kanki* (歓喜). It is a *discipline to experience true joy.

II

How to Control Our Mind and Body through Yoga
- A key to good use and care of the mind and body

Three components of our body

To stay healthy, we must always keep correct posture and correct actions in mind. Correct posture means having a natural body, and correct actions means moving naturally. A semi-healthy person has some distortion or twist. In yoga, the practice of maintaining the correct posture and movement is called *āsana*.

The body consists of three components: muscles, bones, and internal organs. When these three work in smooth cooperation, we can maintain correct posture and correct movement. When their cooperation is abnormal, body movement and posture will be abnormal. The cooperation of these three is successful when each component maintains its characteristics, that is, when muscles are flexible, bones are hard, and internal organs maintain their elasticity.

Muscles stretch and contract. The stronger each of these functions, the more flexible the muscles are. This means that muscles need both stimuli of stretching and contracting. Because usual muscle movements are contracting stimuli, stretching stimuli give the muscles a rest. That is why we feel easier to be sitting than standing, and easier to be lying down than sitting.

In yoga as well, there is more training for muscle stretching than muscle contracting. What yoga calls 'training to relax the body' is the training of stretching muscles. To train muscle contraction, we can practise putting momentary strength into the whole body.

What is more important about muscles is that they lose their flexibility when not used, and they become stiff when the same stimulus is applied repeatedly. And these kinds of functions of muscles affect bones and internal organs. For this reason, sports which are said to be good for health are those that use the whole body. Jogging and swimming are recommended because they are activities involving the whole body.

Partial use of muscles makes them stiff and causes distortion. At the same time, it can also cause skeletal distortion. This is because the bones become malnourished. When muscles become stiff, bones become anaemic and weak.

Muscular and skeletal distortion result in the incorrect positioning of the internal organs. Only when muscles and bones are strong, each internal organ will stay where it should be and maintain its normal function.

Uddīyāna is the key to a natural body

So, how can we maintain correct movement and posture? In other words, what is the key to having a natural body? It is to enhance the power of *tanden (hara)*. This means *'uddīyāna'* in yoga.

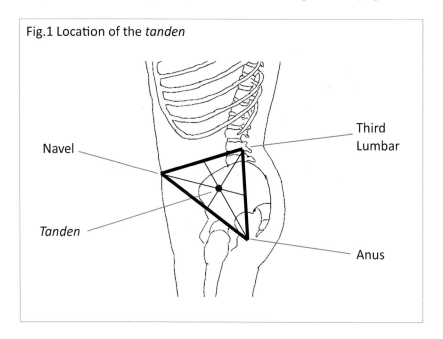

Fig.1 Location of the *tanden*

Navel

Tanden

Third Lumbar

Anus

The *tanden* is the central point of the body, both mechanically and physiologically. It is the centre of a triangle formed by the following three points: the third lumbar, navel and anus. So, that is about 5 cm[6] below the navel in height, and inside the body.

From the physiological aspect, the *tanden* is the centre for balancing the autonomic nerves and body fluids. In yoga, we train our body to be in a state where strength is focused only in the *tanden* with other parts relaxed. This state is called 'Upper body relaxed, lower body powerful' or 'Head cool, feet warm'. In this state, the mental and physical abilities are maximised. The opposite state is the so-called 'hot-headed' state. All the physical training of yoga and the lifestyle based on yoga are for acquiring this state of 'Upper body relaxed, lower body powerful'.

In order to enhance the *tanden*'s power, we must relax the upper body, apply strength to the lower body and tighten the anal muscles. To do this, we need to open the chest, bring both shoulder blades closer to the spine, and lower the pelvis. Also, we should put strength into the big toes and inner side of the knees, and relax the shoulders, neck and hands. Then the anal muscles will tighten naturally. We need to straighten the back of the neck and breathe deeply.

The above explanation is for the static posture, but the principle is the same in movement. And if this is applied to all actions in daily life, it will lead to mental stability. On the contrary, when we are in an unstable posture, we are in an abnormally tense state, which causes our mind to be unbalanced.

Please keep in mind that, even if you are in a life-or-death situation, tightening your anal muscles may save your life. Many people become startled or panic in such a situation and end up

---

[6] The reader will notice two different measurements in Page 40 and 52. The translator does not know Masahiro Oki's intention about this difference in the original Japanese book. Therefore, the difference is also kept in this translation.

doing the opposite. Tightening the anal muscles leads to enhanced stability.

The correct way of standing

A natural standing posture is taken when we stand with our feet our own hip-width apart. At the same time, we need to consciously stretch the back of our legs, lower the pelvis, stretch the back of the torso and pull the chin in. Then, the whole body will stand upright, and the back of the neck will stretch.

When you exhale, breathe deeply in a way that naturally raises the ribs. Keep the head high as if pushing the sky, ground the centre of gravity towards the arches of the soles of the feet, spread the chest sideways, and allow the shoulders to hang. At this time, slightly pull the hips backwards and tighten the lower back muscles. Of course, tighten the anal muscles.

When you stand in this way and your breathing is easy, you can say you stand in a correct posture. If your breathing is uneasy, it is because you are standing incorrectly.

For details, please see Fig.2. If you stand following the basics above, as well as according to your mental and physical condition, you will be manifesting a natural body. When you are tense, take a deep breath to relax. Consciously try to smile. The point is to perform the opposite of the negative state of your *mind-heart.

The key point in the correct way of walking

To walk correctly, you need to have the correct stride that suits you. This should be the stride you take when you are standing correctly, gradually leaning forwards and finally taking your first

Fig.2 The correct way of standing

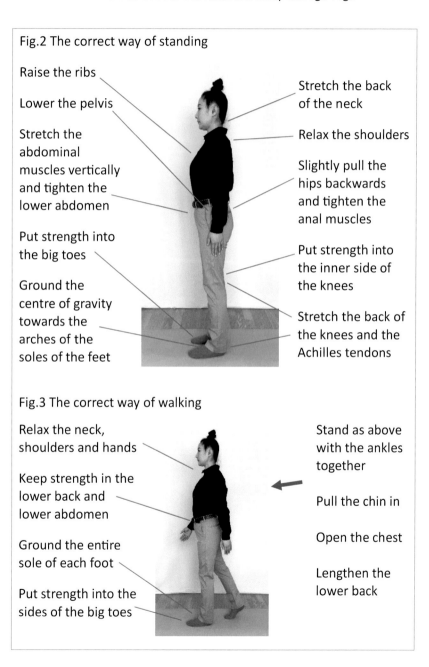

Raise the ribs

Lower the pelvis

Stretch the abdominal muscles vertically and tighten the lower abdomen

Put strength into the big toes

Ground the centre of gravity towards the arches of the soles of the feet

Stretch the back of the neck

Relax the shoulders

Slightly pull the hips backwards and tighten the anal muscles

Put strength into the inner side of the knees

Stretch the back of the knees and the Achilles tendons

Fig.3 The correct way of walking

Relax the neck, shoulders and hands

Keep strength in the lower back and lower abdomen

Ground the entire sole of each foot

Put strength into the sides of the big toes

Stand as above with the ankles together

Pull the chin in

Open the chest

Lengthen the lower back

step. Once you know your stride, the rest is not so difficult. First, try not to make any noise. Also, in the same way as you stand, put strength into the big toes, but not into the sides of the little toes.

Appearances aside, high heels are not desirable footwear, because they contract the Achilles tendons. People who wear high heels should try to stretch the Achilles tendons as often as possible, for example by standing on their toes (heels off the floor) on some stairs.

Nowadays, we rarely have a chance to wear wooden sandals (*geta* [7]) or straw sandals (*waraji* [8]). However, because these encourage the wearer to put strength into the big toes, they are good footwear in this respect.

As any movement and posture should be performed with strength in the *tanden*, we, when walking, must try to keep strength in the lower back and lower abdomen, relax the neck, shoulders and hands, stretch the Achilles tendons, and make sure that the entire sole of each foot is grounded.

People who work mainly with their hands or brain must consciously put strength into their lower body. The balance that yoga teaches is to use what we don't often use.

The correct way of sitting on the floor

No matter how you sit, please relax your upper body. That is, relax your shoulders, neck, and hands. Put strength into your lower body, namely, your lower back, abdomen, and legs. How to sit in *seiza* [9] is illustrated in the next page. Please refer to Fig.4.

---

[7] and [8] Both are traditional Japanese footwear with a strap that separates the big toe from the other toes.

[9] Sitting down in Japanese style with the buttocks on top of the ankles.

Fig.4 The correct way of sitting on the floor

Raise the ribs

Stretch the abdominal muscles vertically

Tighten the lower abdomen and put strength in the *tanden*

Lift the head up towards the ceiling

Line up the ear and shoulder vertically on each side

Pull the hips backwards and tighten the anal muscles

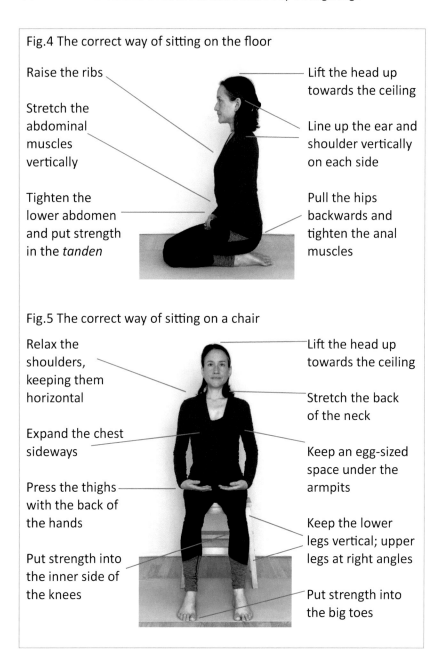

Fig.5 The correct way of sitting on a chair

Relax the shoulders, keeping them horizontal

Expand the chest sideways

Press the thighs with the back of the hands

Put strength into the inner side of the knees

Lift the head up towards the ceiling

Stretch the back of the neck

Keep an egg-sized space under the armpits

Keep the lower legs vertical; upper legs at right angles

Put strength into the big toes

The correct way of sitting on a chair

When we use a chair, the basic points are the same as those already explained. Do not rest your body on the backrest. Open your chest in the same way as when you sit in *seiza*. Refer to Fig.5.

The key point in the correct way of standing up

By consciously performing various daily-life movements as yoga teaches, you will become healthy both physically and mentally. And that will also give a happy feeling to other people around you.

When you stand up from *seiza*, first take a breath and keep strength in the *tanden*. Also, straighten your back, pull your chin in, and look straight forwards.

Then, as you inhale, relax your shoulders while keeping them horizontal, and lift your hips. At that time, tuck the toes under, place the centre of gravity towards the big toes, and stand up without making a sound. What is forbidden in this series of actions is doing in reaction. Don't use reactive force at all. Refer to Fig.6.

When you sit down, do the same actions in reverse order while exhaling.

It is incorrect to stand with your eyes looking downwards or with your back rounded. This doesn't look good either.

Yogic marathon running that emphasises balance

What I mention here as 'marathon' is not competitive running. I mean jogging for wellbeing which anyone can do easily and for free. Jogging is very popular nowadays, but is it really good for anyone?

Fig.6 The correct way of standing up

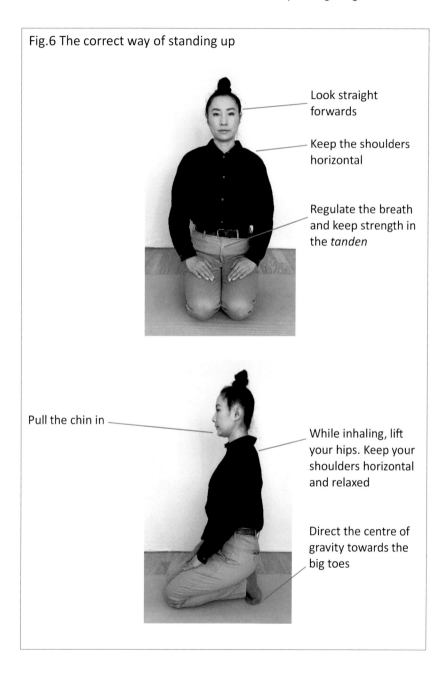

Look straight forwards

Keep the shoulders horizontal

Regulate the breath and keep strength in the *tanden*

Pull the chin in

While inhaling, lift your hips. Keep your shoulders horizontal and relaxed

Direct the centre of gravity towards the big toes

It depends on how you do it. In yogic marathon running, it is important to jog at your own pace, and according to your mental and physical condition.

If you compete with other people, run with a bad posture or push too hard, it may bring abnormalities to your body. It is a mistake to assume that marathon running is always a health regime.

Running is an exercise for the whole body, but it particularly stresses the heart, lungs and legs. Those who have a problem in any of these areas cannot overdo it. Conversely, for people in good health, the more they run the stronger they can make the functions of their heart, lungs and legs.

The above is what is commonly said about marathon running. Then, what is the attitude of yoga towards marathon running?

Yoga puts importance on balance. In the case of marathon running as well, you must devise a way to create balance. That is to say, instead of just running, you should run forwards, then backwards, and so on. Running backwards allows you to rest the muscles you use for running forwards and prevent partial fatigue.

Next, regarding how to run, basically you must use the whole body. Without bending your upper body, relax your chest and above, lower your shoulders, keep your hips and upper body stable, and move forwards from your hips. Breathe rhythmically, breathing in, in, out, out, and so on.

In addition to the usual way of running, please: ①run sideways like a crab; ②run crossing the legs and twisting the hips; ③run on tiptoes; ④run raising the thighs high; ⑤run as if kicking the buttocks with the heels; ⑥run with big strides; ⑦run while waving your hands up, down, left and right, or rotating the arms, and so on.

Furthermore, you can add some exercises for the shoulder blades, neck and eyes; for instance, jog for 20 steps with your shoulder blades close together and your head and eyes turning right, and then for 20 steps with your head and eyes turning left. It is also good to jog while rotating the eyeballs.

If your right (left) leg is longer, you had better run with more right (left) turns. Also, it is good to run with your longer leg stepping on the higher side of the road.

Regarding how long you should jog, consider it to be the time that you can jog with your shoulder blades close together. This means that the running form should be to keep the chest open and the shoulder blades closed. If you cannot maintain this form, you will be overdoing it.

After the yogic marathon, which makes your body warm up, sweat and improve blood circulation, please take a cold bath to tighten the blood vessels. This is effective from the perspective of the balance between tension and relaxation of the whole body.

In the current jogging boom, people are concerned about distance, time duration and speed. But yoga focuses on balance. You can see that just by reading what I have described above. The key to yogic jogging is to try various ways of running and combine them well.

Importance of breathing training

We can live for about 60 days if we don't eat anything and only drink water. However, we will die if we stop breathing for any longer than three minutes. Therefore, it can be said that breathing is our life.

Since ancient times, 'breath' has been regarded as very important, and it has been thought that there is a significant connection between breathing and living. In the Japanese language, the word 'iki-suru', which means to breathe, has become the word *'iki-ru'*, which means to live. Also, realising that long and deep breaths are good for health, *'nagai-iki'*, which means long breath, has become *'naga-iki'*, which means long life.

In this way people gave birth to the thought that breath is life, and so breathing plays the most important role in the function of human life. When breathing stops, not only humans but all living creatures die.

Yogic breathing training has been an experiential study of the physiology and effects of breathing. The key to doing everything correctly is said to be the way of breathing. Let's practise yogic breathing techniques to grasp the key points about life.

As mentioned above, in yoga, breathing is always important. I have said that our posture is good if we can breathe comfortably in that posture. I mean that is deep breathing. In other words, it is 'breath of laughter'.

In general, there are two types of breathing: chest breathing and abdominal breathing. Chest breathing is shallow breathing and easily excites our nerves. In contrast, abdominal breathing is deep breathing, and it enhances the ability to relax and makes the pulse and blood pressure stable. In this state, we can deal with anything in a calm feeling like when laughing, without being nervous. We usually mix these two types of breathing, which is called in yoga 'complete breathing' or 'whole body breathing'.

By training, we improve our breathing from chest breathing to abdominal breathing, that is to say, from shallow breathing to deep breathing, which uses the whole body where the strength is naturally put in the lower abdomen with the shoulders and neck relaxed, as happens in laughter. This training is called *'prānāyāma'*. Deep abdominal breathing is practised as follows:

First, bring both shoulder blades as close together as possible. Naturally, your chest opens. Think of your body as a balloon, inhale with your whole body, and exhale while pulling your abdomen in. The key to exhaling is to put more effort into your abdominal muscles. It will not be so difficult. However, you must be able to do it naturally, both when studying and when working. The reason is that abdominal breathing is desirable especially when the mind and body are tense, such as when working or studying.

Abdominal breathing calms the nerves and promotes blood circulation throughout the whole body. As this helps the function of the heart, the abdomen is also said to be the second heart. This means that you are also doing light physical exercise.

Moreover, when you breathe very deeply, your upper body relaxes and lower body becomes stronger, and so this breathing is also called 'feet breathing'. It is said in yoga, 'A true person breathes with his feet'. The feet, which help the function of the heart, are the third heart.

I have said that chest breathing easily makes the nerves restless and excited. Our daily life is full of stress. In other words, we are living a daily life where we cannot help but get excited by stimuli. This makes us rely on chest breathing. Therefore, it is necessary to consciously change the way we breathe from shallow breathing to deep breathing.

Health method through yogic breathing exercises

(1) *Sītalī Prānāyāma* to purify the blood

From the perspective of the blood, illness is a sign of poor blood quality, poor blood flow, or both. When blood flow is poor and also its quality is poor, the body is almost close to death. Some people are even partially dead. This means that our body will be dying slowly step by step if we don't use our whole body in a well-balanced way to always maintain clean blood. For that reason,

Sītalī Prāṇāyāma is an important method, which helps to purify the blood.

▪ Method

First, roll your tongue like a tube and stick it out a little between your lips. Inhale through your mouth, making a sucking sound, and hold your breath for as long as possible but without forcing. Then exhale quietly through both nostrils. This can be practised while sitting, standing or walking. About 15 minutes can be a good target. This is a breathing method that you can do whenever you want to, such as when you are waiting for the bus or train.

This breathing technique not only purifies the blood but also relieves thirst and hunger. It can also heal chronic dyspepsia, inflammation and other types of fever, pulmonary tuberculosis, and so on. After a long period of practising this technique, the blood will be so purified that one would not be affected by the deadly poison of a snake. Adding *Kumbhaka* to this breathing technique is called 'imitating a snake'. Also, by continuing to practise this technique, you will gain perseverance and, for instance, be able to withstand lack of food or air.

(2) *Kumbhaka* to enhance the power of unification

Kumbhaka means 'retaining breath'. When do we retain our breath? Please think. It is when we lift something, focus our mind on something, endure pain, and so on. In each case, with the breath retained, the power of the whole body is unified in the lower abdomen. Our power to perform *Kumbhaka* indicates our lung capacity, and the lung capacity indicates our vital force.

▪ Method

You can sit or stand. Take a full breath, exhale a little and retain your breath. At that time, tighten your anal muscles strongly, detach your mind from all things in the outside world, and bring it to the point between the eyebrows or to the *tanden*.

Beginners had better practise focusing their mind on the *tanden* because, if they concentrate on the point between the eyebrows without enough preparation, the centre of gravity in their body will rise up. So, please concentrate on the *tanden*.

The *tanden*, which appears many times in this book, does not have a fixed shape like that of a nose or ear. It is located in the centre of the triangle that connects the navel, the third lumbar and the anus. It is an intangible point which makes you feel power in the depth of the abdomen, at *Heso-shita-san-zun* (three *suns*[10] below the navel), when you put strength into your big toes and tighten your anal muscles.

In order to put strength in the *tanden* and unify the mind and body, we have to tighten our anal muscles. However, when we feel loose or reluctant and the *tanden*'s power is weak, the anus is also loosely open. If someone is drowning and their anus is open, it is unlikely that they will survive.

This breathing technique can be called 'a breathing method to enhance energy'.

(3) *Sītkārī* to get out of sleepiness

In yoga, it is said that we don't need to sleep for more than six hours. Overeating is the greatest cause of sleepiness. If we eat too much, our internal organs will get tired and we will need a lot of oxygen, which will make us sleepy immediately. It takes longer to recover from fatigue of the internal organs than muscular fatigue. So, if we ignore it and continue such eating habits, we may end up with serious illness.

---

[10] *Sun* is a Japanese traditional unit to measure length. One *sun* is about 3 cm, which makes three *suns* about 9 cm. '*Heso-shita-san-zun*' is a traditional expression which describes the position of the *tanden* and is often used to mean the *tanden* itself.

It is possible that we eat or drink too much when socialising, but I suggest that we don't eat the next day.

Yoga emphasises balance and tells us to always have the opposite stimulation. When the opposite stimulation is given, the symptom disappears.

• Method

To avoid sleepiness, first roll your tongue and lightly attach its tip to the back of your upper jaw. Then open your mouth slightly and inhale gradually from there. If your tongue hurts, you can put your tongue between your lips and inhale through the gap. Inhale while making a sound and exhale through your nose.

This method is effective not only for sleepiness but also for maintaining beauty and strengthening the body. It can also relieve hunger and thirst and eliminate laziness. You can practise this technique while sitting or walking.

Furthermore, I often see people drinking juices and stimulating drinks, tempted by the taste. However, if you repeat such a thing, you will not only feel sleepy, but your liver will be weakened, and your nerves won't work properly. Please try to control your body.

(4) A breathing technique to help the brain work clearly

The cranial nerves work most clearly when:

① Sufficient nutrients such as oxygen, lactic acid, glutamic acid, vitamins B, C and E are available enough with low levels of waste products,

② The mind and body are relaxed, not tired, or stiffened,

③ The excitatory nerves and inhibitory nerves are antagonistically working well,

④ The mind is focused on something you are interested in or care about, and so on.

If the neck, which acts as a pipe to the brain, is stiff, blood circulation in the brain will become poorer. It can even cause a headache. Therefore, it is also necessary to keep your shoulders and neck flexible. The breathing technique described next will help you replenish oxygen, improve blood circulation in the brain by relaxing the mind and body, and concentrate your attention. Please practise as follows:

▪ Method

Sit with your back straight and place your palms down on your thighs. In this posture, move only your head rhythmically back and forth. When the head moves forwards, make your chin almost touch the chest, and when it moves backwards, make the back of the head almost touch your back. Repeat this several times.

Also, when tilting your head backwards, take a deep breath through both nostrils with a whooshing sound. When tilting your head forwards, open your mouth slightly and exhale, making a hissing sound between your teeth. Move your head back and forth in this way ten times, in a rhythmic manner like the pendulum of a clock. When that is done, rest for a while. Then repeat 10 more times and take a rest. With this technique, be careful not to move the whole body except the head. And it is necessary to practise this while focusing your mind on something.

The basis of a yogic diet is a small meal of diverse foods

In yoga, diet is as important as breathing for mental and physical health. Yoga teaches 'Make your food your medicine'. Many people are unaware that it is only natural to eat foods containing the nutrients that meet their needs in the correct quantities.

Medical drugs have side effects. It is said that the more effective the medical drugs, the stronger their side effects. However, when we take an appropriate amount at the right time, they work brilliantly. Good doctors are excellent at adjusting the amount of medicine.

Young children, adolescents, old people and so on—as different people need different diets, everybody should eat according to their needs. If you think of food as medicine, you will understand that you shouldn't eat or drink too much. Taking too much medicine can lead to death. Similarly, over-eating and over-drinking can lead to poor health.

In short, a yogic meal is a small meal of diverse foods. The energy left in the body by overeating does not lead to improving physical strength but becomes energy to cause illness. Ideally, we should maximise our digestive, absorptive, and excretory capacities and eat when we are ready to eat.

In recent years, the life expectancy of Japanese people has become the highest in the world for both men and women. The reason is often said to be the rich variety in the Japanese diet. No other ethnic group eats as diversely as the Japanese. Japanese

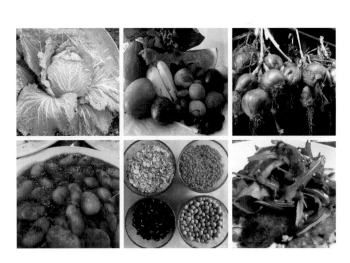

A yogic diet is based on a small meal of diverse foods

people eat meat as well as fish, and things from the sea as well as from the mountains. Food is cooked in various styles such as Japanese, Western, Chinese and so on. This exemplifies very well what yoga means by 'diverse foods'. However, when it comes to 'eating a small meal', the number of people who fail to do so is increasing nowadays.

It is important to have a balance between taking things in and moving things out. Many people are concerned about eating, but not many people put importance on eliminating. Many people disregard that their ability for excretion may be declining and neglect to maintain and improve it. This increases the residual energy in the body and is not good for it. You could say that a good time to eat is also a good time for your body's excretory function.

The key to good dietary habits is not to enjoy the fullness of our stomach, but to enjoy its emptiness. In other words, we should value a small meal.

So, what can you do to improve your dietary habits?

First of all, the basic question is what, how much, and how to eat. However, this depends on each individual and is not for others to teach. It is important to consult your own body. When you are excited or nervous, you will not get the correct answer. You should follow your dietary needs when you are in a calm and relaxed state.

In yoga, we follow a 'natural diet' to awaken to our body's actual needs. A natural diet consists of two aspects: whole food and raw food. A whole food diet means: for example, when we eat vegetables, we eat the leaves, stems and roots. When we eat fish, we eat the skin, flesh and bones. Raw food means uncooked food.

As an even stricter measure, we reduce food or do fasting. By reducing or fasting, we can reflect through our experience how unhealthy our diet used to be, and we can smoothly shift to a diet consisting of smaller meals.

How can you practise a diet of 'diverse foods'? It is to eat by combining foods from the river and sea, foods which warm your body and foods which cool it (such as brown rice and wheat), foods that contract your body and foods that loosen it (such as salt and sugar), animal protein and vegetable protein, and so on.

By eating like this, you can take good things for your whole body. Don't eat with a partial purpose such as eating because something is good for your liver or good for your eyes. You should aim at a well-balanced diet so that all the parts of your mind and body can fully exert their functions.

Whether a food is good for you or not can be determined by how it is excreted from the body. If it doesn't suit your body, you may have constipation, or if it is extremely unsuitable, you may have diarrhoea. Also, even with suitable foods, if the amount is too large, the body will feel heavy and dull, which will make you sleepy from the morning. On the contrary, if you wake up feeling clear in mind and light in body and you want to move and work, then your diet is right for you.

Create balance in your diet

I have said that the dietary principle is a small meal of diverse foods. I will explain a little more why diverse foods are important.

There are two types of food: one that cools the body and the other one that warms the body. Foods that cool the body are called yin[11], and foods that warm the body are called yang[12]. Yang foods are those that grow in the sea rather than on land, and,

---

[11] and [12] In Eastern philosophy, the two great opposite forces are thought to be complementarily working to make up all phenomena in the universe. Yin is the expansive force, and yang is the contractive force.

regarding plants, grow in the shade rather than in the sun and are the root rather than the part growing above ground. These foods have the stronger ability to absorb sunlight and therefore warm our body. In yoga, we give importance to foods that warm the body.

Blood acidifies when you use the body. So, in order to maintain a weak alkaline state in your body, please make sure not to miss alkaline foods. However, the human body is designed to return to a weak alkaline state when the blood acidifies, and so you would not need to be so nervous about whether the food is acidic or alkaline. It will be good enough if you are careful not to take an unbalanced diet.

Regarding breakfast and lunch, because you do activity after these meals, the blood acidifies. As a rule, please take alkaline foods. Regarding supper, because you are going to sleep after the meal and so the blood alkalises, you can eat meat or fish that are acidic foods. To avoid the ingested meat or fish rotting in the body, please take vegetables which contain minerals at the same time.

Don't eat anything just before going to bed. Eating raises your body temperature, which disturbs your deep sleep.

The universe provides food for each season so that we can create balance in our diet. For instance, we can eat in spring what grows in spring, or eat in summer what grows in summer. Nowadays, seasonality in food is lost, but it makes sense to eat seasonal food. We are to eat what cools the body in the summer months and what warms it in the winter ones.

One thing you should keep in mind is to avoid eating what will rot in your body. Meat is often eaten just before it rots because it is tastier then. However, you should not eat a lot. In contrast, smoked or dried fish works as a detoxifier.

By the way, needless to say, meals are not only a source of nourishment, but they are also a source of enjoyment. This is often overlooked at first glance, but it is important. An insipid meal tends to be unbalanced, and a pleasant meal balanced. A meal should be considered as medicine, but what makes it different is that it is an enjoyable cultural event.

Unlike animals, we humans have a *mind-heart, so we enjoy taking a meal. That is good for nutrition. No matter how much raw vegetables with live elements have the effect of strengthening the internal organs, bringing much oxygen into the body and enhancing the ability of neutralisation and excretion, always eating raw vegetables will rather create an adverse effect for people who tend to have a colder body constitution.

The basics of a good diet are to not eat too much and to eat a wide variety of foods prepared by applying different cooking methods. Those who can do that will not have to pay particular attention to their diet.

How to drink alcohol

Alcohol is said to be 'the best among all medicines' and has been loved as a friend of mankind since ancient times. However, the more effective the medicine, the more we must be careful.

Compared with other foods and drinks, alcohol is absorbed more quickly in the gastrointestinal tract and reaches the liver faster. Its breakdown puts a heavy burden on the liver. Therefore, it is beneficial to drink while eating so that it can be absorbed slowly. In other words, don't forget the accompanying snacks. Also, if you drink with an empty stomach, absorption will be faster, so it is a good idea to eat a light meal before drinking.

Some alcoholic beverages, such as whisky, have high alcohol content, while others, such as beer, have weak alcohol content.

The stronger the alcohol, the more important it is to drink slowly while eating snacks or taking a meal.

As I am not one who dislikes alcohol, I drink whisky like other people. I usually dilute it with hot water. Traveling around the world, I think Japanese people are not so tolerant to alcohol. A strong drink like whisky, which originated in a foreign country and is familiar to Westerners with a good physique, can't be drunk in the same way by the Japanese. The style of drinking straight in one gulp isn't worth admiring. It suits Japanese people to dilute it with water. At its core, yoga teaches that we should not imitate others. In other words, it is a teaching that every person should live just as they are. So, Japanese people should drink like Japanese people.

Also, alcohol is a source of energy. Drinking too much can lead to obesity. However, what we must be more careful about is that some people become resistant to alcohol (become slower to get drunk), increase their drinking, and eventually become unable to live without alcohol. In short, they become addicted to it. To prevent this, drink with a stable mind. If you drink to get out of stress or in place of sleeping pills, it will cause your body to be out of balance. On the other hand, drinking at festive events is your enjoyment and will have a positive effect on your mind and body.

A hangover occurs when you cannot help but drink more than you should. In that case, you need to take water first. Then, by refraining from alcohol in order to rest organs such as the liver, you will feel better. It is out of the question to cure a hangover by drinking alcohol further. It is a deception.

Cure imbalances of the mind with yogic reverse thinking

So far, I have talked about what yoga teaches from the physical aspect. Now let's talk about the mental aspect.

An unbalanced mind can also cause impairment of health. We tend to think of the mind and body as separate things. But humans cannot be easily divided in that way. The balance of emotions, intellect and desires is a major factor in good health because the mind and body function using the same brain, nerves, blood and organs. When you feel depressed, do you have an appetite? When you are having fun, don't you feel lighter? When you have anxiety, you may not be able to sleep. The mind directly affects the body, and the body directly affects the mind.

In yoga, we regard 'the mind and body as one'. Therefore, in yoga there is no training only for the mind or only for the body. In my *dōjō*, we train at a ratio of seven for the mind and three for the body for mental and physical health.

From the point of view that the mind and body are one, it is unlikely that those who have been cultivating their mind are physically weak. This is impossible indeed. It is because, if we give a good stimulus to our mind, it should also give a good stimulus to our body. Mental training leads to physical training. Conversely, training that is good for the body is also good for the mind.

Then, what is a good state of mind? It is a state of peace.

When the mind is in this state, there is no tension in the mind or body. It is a peaceful *mind-heart with which you can feel joy in everything. It is not a state of lethargy or apathy. It is a state in which there is no bias in desires or emotions. In short, you are a 'free' person. There is no attachment or bias, and there is stability. In that state, you are fully living as you are.

How can you get into that state? This is what this book is consistently pursuing. But for now, please keep the following in mind:

• When you think "I want", think "I don't need",
• When you think "It is unlikely that I can do", think "I may be able to do",

- When you think "I don't like", think "I am grateful",
- When you think "It's okay", think "It might not be", and so on.

It is a good idea to always give yourself this kind of opposite stimulation. In this way, you can be well-balanced, feeling good whether it is sunny or rainy.

Even when you are nervous in an important interview and you think the other person is great, think the opposite as well. Smiling inwardly and regarding the situation as less serious often brings about a good result.

Regarding intellectual matters, try to distinguish what you understand and what you don't understand.

Many people try to figure out what they don't understand. It is unnecessary. The more you forcibly try to understand what you don't know, the more misunderstandings will increase, and the more delusions or illusions will arise. It is all right to understand what you can understand and to not understand what you cannot understand. This distinction keeps the naturalness of your mind.

For example, let's say you have had a heartbreak. Trying to know or understand why that has happened will create misunderstandings and delusions. The other party doesn't really know why they have come to dislike you. Even if you find out in detail, your mental balance will not be restored. In short, you had better leave things you don't understand, without affirming or denying, and wait until you can understand them. This is called 'leaving your fate in Nature's hands'.

The yogic way of controlling mind and body

We are not in a peaceful, balanced state of mind all day long. Someone who can do this is a saint, a free person whose *busshō* is enlightened, namely a Buddha. Even those who have practised yoga to some extent can get caught up in their desires, feel disappointed with failures and make mistakes in their judgments. Here, let's think about how to control such situations using breathing techniques and physical exercises.

(1) <u>When you are frustrated</u> (Fig.7)
The cause of frustration varies from person to person. Some people may get frustrated by missing a train and waiting for the next 10 minutes even though they won't be particularly late for work. On the other hand, there are those who may not mind at all standing in a long queue to buy a train ticket. However, everyone would have some cause for frustration. When you are frustrated, your stomach pit and neck are usually stiff. So, you need to loosen muscles in those areas. Bathing is also effective.

(2) <u>When you are angry</u> (Fig.8)
The cause is clearer than when you are frustrated. It is often caused by the actions of other people against your will. About this state, one says 'the blood rises', which cannot be good for your health. Blood pressure also jumps up.

When you are angry, the muscles of your stomach pit, neck, and back are stiff. Relax those areas and do exercises such as twisting or bending the body. At the same time, put strength into your legs and hips in order to lower the centre of gravity of your body.

If your body is not in a state that easily leads to anger, you will not get angry even when you want to get angry. You can say that this is a well-balanced state, that is, a healthy state.

(3) <u>When you are unhappy</u> (Fig.9)
When you are unhappy, your chest muscles are shrunk and your back muscles are stiff so that you have a hunched posture. Exercises to fully open your chest will help this problem. It is also a good

Fig.7 When you are frustrated

Breathe deeply
while shaking
your body

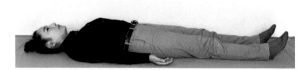

Fig.8 When you are angry

1 Move your legs together up and down

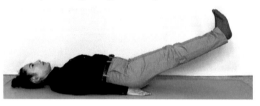

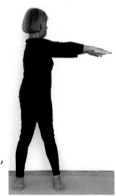

2 While inhaling, extend your
arms forwards. While exhaling,
twist your body

3 While exhaling, bend your body sideways

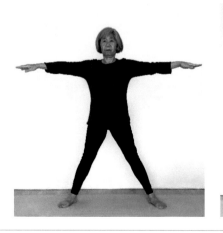

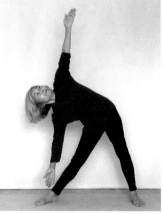

Fig.9 When you are unhappy

1 Fish Pose

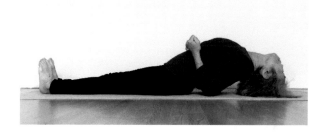

2 Arch Pose (Wheel Pose)

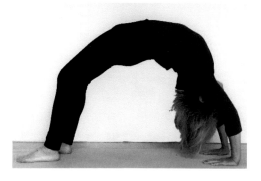

4 Headstand Pose

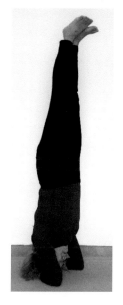

3 Breathe deeply in a good posture

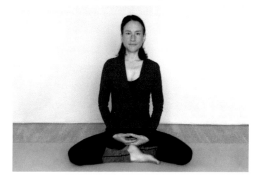

idea to stretch your chest, put strength into your lower abdomen and breathe deeply and quietly.

For a change of mood, drinking alcohol and having fun are effective. But please keep in mind that these inexpensive exercises I have mentioned here are also very effective.

(4) When you feel unsettled (Fig.10)

The shoulders, neck and hands are tense, and the legs and hips are loose. Therefore, bring strength to the abdomen by stomping in a Japanese sumo wrestler's way or jumping like a rabbit in a squatting position. Also, if you put strength into your feet, stretch your chest well and breathe quietly and deeply, you will calm yourself down.

A further way to make your mind stable is to confirm the facts. A proverb says, 'Flowers are red, and willows are green'. All you have to do is make sure that red is red and green is green. The key to not getting upset is to acquire the ability to feel the truth, see the truth and think as it is. When you feel unsettled, your upper body is too tense. So, you must first loosen it.

(5) When you are startled (Fig.11)

When you are startled, you are putting strength into the little toe side of your foot, the lower back is loose, and the shoulders and neck are stiffened. To get out of this state, put strength into your big toes and lower back, relax your shoulders, and breathe deeply. Of course, it is abdominal breathing.

(6) When you are lacking energy (Fig.12)

When you are lacking energy despite having nothing wrong with you, your lower back is stiff, your neck is weak, and your chin sticks out. So, stretch your chest, pull your chin in, stretch your back, and do strong abdominal breathing. The key to breathing like this is to

Fig.10 When you feel unsettled

1 Stomp in a Japanese *sumō* wrestler's way

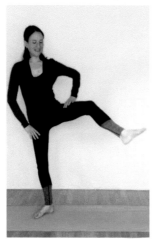

2 Jump like a rabbit in a squatting position

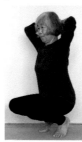

3 Breathe deeply with your legs bent halfway and hips lowered

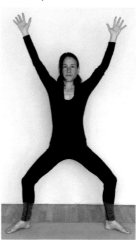

Fig.11 When you are startled

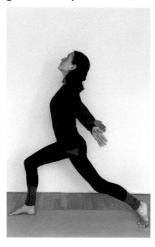

(left) Take one big step forwards and inhale

(right) Put strength into your big toes. Stretch your chest. Do quiet abdominal breathing

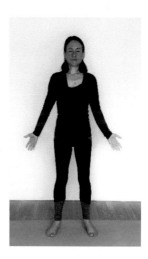

Fig.12 When you are lacking energy

1 Stretch your chest, pull your chin in

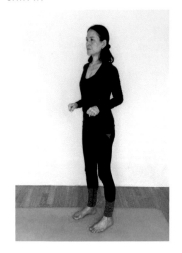

While exhaling, move your fists fast forwards and backwards

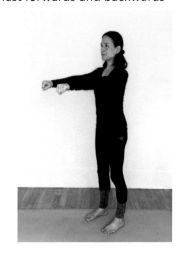

2 While inhaling, lift your heels

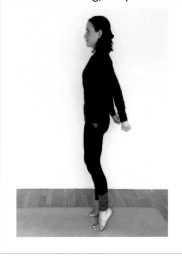

While exhaling, bend your legs and thrust your fists forwards

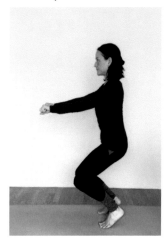

Fig.13 When hysteria occurs

1 Lift your chest
and hips with your
elbows and drop
them all at once

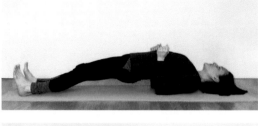

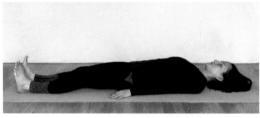

2 With your feet together
and arms L-shaped, raise
the hips and move them up
and down

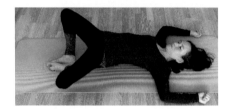

hold your breath in for a while (*Kumbhaka*) and then exhale all at once in a self-motivating tone.

(7) When hysteria occurs (Fig.13)
The occurrence of hysteria can depend on personality, but it is more or less common among women. In this case, the pelvis is tightened. Please do such exercises as to turn your knees outwards and open your chest. These have a good effect on the pelvis as well.

(8) When you become nervous (Fig.14)
If you are not used to being at the centre of attention at big events,

Fig.14 When you become nervous

1 Bend and extend your legs
repeatedly

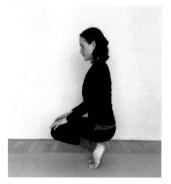
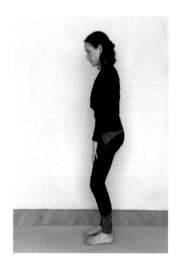

2 While inhaling, bend down, and while exhaling, stretch up

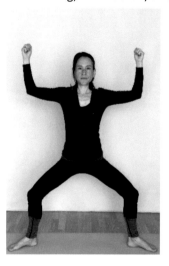
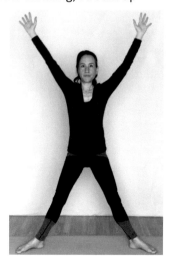

you will most likely be nervous and let the occasion pass by without really experiencing it. Even if you hear such advice as "Think of the audience as lined-up watermelons", it will not work easily. Then, you can do the following exercises:

Relax your shoulders and neck, and flex and extend your knees. Put strength into your feet and lower back and exhale strongly.

(9) <u>When distracting thoughts and delusions occur</u> (Fig.15)
In any case, the neck is stiff. A headstand will work best, but it will also be effective to rotate the neck or flex and extend it.

Fig.15 When distracting thoughts and delusions occur

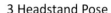
3 Headstand Pose

1 Raise your shoulders up and down repeatedly

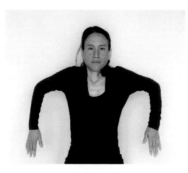

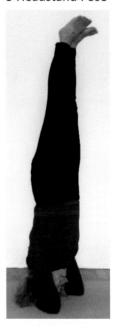

2 Rotate your neck

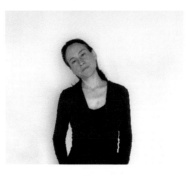

(10) <u>When you cannot make a decision</u>
Let's put strength into the feet and lower back and laugh out loud. You can then make up your mind without hesitation and may even come up with a good idea. When you think about something, make sure that you are thinking with a clear mind. You should make a decision within the range of resources you have in order to guide your judgement.

(11) <u>When you don't feel like doing anything</u> (Fig.16)
There is no doubt that your Achilles tendons are contracted. Pull your chin in, stretch your chest, and stretch the back muscles of your legs. It is also effective to put strength into your feet and lower back and twist your arms while exhaling deeply.

(12) <u>When you are in trouble</u>
The kinds of trouble mentioned here refer to the following cases:
① When you have bought too much or have eaten a lot,
② When you are being overly persistent,
③ When you cannot focus on work or study but just walk around.
    In all cases, too much energy remains in your body. A few minutes of exercise is not enough. You must take the plunge and move a lot to dissipate your energy.

Health tips for the semi-healthy

(1) <u>How to relieve shoulder stiffness</u>
If you wrongly use or cultivate your mind and body in daily life, you will fall into a so-called semi-healthy state. Now let's see the main symptoms of this condition.
    Stiffness is caused when you put unnecessary extra force in that part of the body or use it forcibly. Due to this, the muscles hold

Fig.16 When you don't feel like doing anything

1 Take a big step forwards and stretch the Achilles tendon of the back leg. Place your hands on your lower back and inhale. While exhaling, bring the front leg back. Then do the same with the other leg

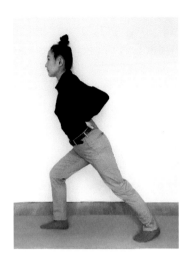

2 While exhaling, rotate the arms internally.

While inhaling, rotate them externally

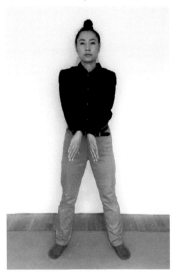

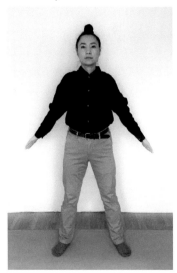

tension and blood circulation becomes poor. Shoulder stiffness relates to the following three factors:

① The posture is abnormal. If your lower body, especially your lower back, is weak, your shoulders will try to make up for it with extra tension.

② If there is something wrong with the internal organs, the related parts will be stressed in an attempt to cover the function. For example, if your stomach is in a bad condition, you will unintentionally lower your left shoulder. If you have an abnormality in your teeth, your shoulders will be stiff. Stiffness of the right shoulder relates to the liver, gallbladder and so on. Stiffness of the left shoulder relates to the heart, stomach, pancreas and so on.

③ Whenever you are in a state of mental abnormality, tension, excitement or lethargy, the center of gravity of your body is raised, that is, you are in the 'hot-headed' state. The tension of the shoulders cannot be released. If you reluctantly work or study with irritation, you may get shoulder stiffness.

To loosen shoulder stiffness, you need to relax the shoulder muscles and improve the blood flow. It is good to give acupressure or massage to the upper area of each shoulder blade. This is the muscle group which rises when you shrug your shoulders.

Press that area towards the centre of your abdomen, using your three middle fingers, and gradually increase the pressure. Press the right shoulder side with your left hand and the left shoulder side with your right hand.

In order to relax your shoulders, you can also rotate an extended arm inwardly or outwardly, which is very effective to relieve shoulder stiffness.

However, something like toothache will first need treatment such as tooth extraction.

In the case of ③, the aforementioned exercises for controlling the mind and body are also effective. The best is *Meditation, which will be explained in detail in Chapter 6.

When your shoulders are stiff, focusing solely on massaging them may have the opposite effect of increasing the stiffness (although it will work if the cause is just located there).

(2) How to relieve pain in your back
Pain in your lower or upper back is caused by abnormality in your posture or internal organs.

A person with such pain generally has a hunched spine. This is not because there is something wrong with the spine, but because the spine is pulled to the side which has stiffness. In other words, the condition of the muscles of the lower or upper back is not uniform and is very unbalanced.

If you have a bad posture, your muscles will be unbalanced. If you have abnormalities in your internal organs, they will cause abnormalities in your muscles through your nerves.

In order to recover from these abnormalities, it is necessary to relax the stiff areas, put strength into the loose areas, improve the blood circulation and awaken the paralysed areas.

You should be careful if the spine and hip bones are weak. In this case, stiffness means that the muscles are supporting the weak area, acting like a splint by becoming stiff. It is rather dangerous to apply massage or acupressure in such a situation.

(3) How to relieve a congested nose
A person with a bad nose condition has a twisted neck and poor blood circulation to the nose. This causes inflammation of the mucous membranes of the nose, which can sometimes become infected. A twisted neck is due to an imbalance between the left and right sides of the body. To relieve this nose problem, apply

acupressure to the wings of the nose and exercise the neck by rotating it or moving it back, forth, left and right.

Acupressure on the wings of the nose with the middle fingers will improve the sense of smell, relieve a congested nose or rhinitis, and improve the airways. You can do this as follows:

First rub the palms together 20-30 times to warm them up, and then place the middle fingers on the sides of the wings of the nose. Then, move them up and down quickly along both sides of the nose. This improves blood circulation in the nose and helps to remove congestion. Exhale strongly when you move your fingers upwards, and inhale as necessary.

Then, place your middle fingers firmly next to the sides of the wings and press for 5 seconds while exhaling strongly and continuously. Release your fingers after exhalation. Repeat this about 5 times.

(4) How to alleviate a headache and absent-mindedness

We humans must stimulate our brain as long as we are alive so that the normal function of the brain is constantly maintained. To do this, we need to use our brain and also exercise our body in order for fresh blood to flow into the brain. If we don't, the function of the brain will become dull, and our memory especially will deteriorate.

By the way, there are various types of headaches, and the causes are also diverse. The main causes are lack of sleep, arteriosclerosis, high blood pressure, constipation, overwork, fatigue from studying, and so on. Also, there seem to be many cases caused by stiff neck or shoulders. When you have a headache, the area around your head and lower neck is often stiff. So, you can start alleviating it by thoroughly loosening these parts.

Acupressure is effective for relieving a headache. There are acupressure points that are effective for headaches. The acupressure point at the top of the head is called *Hyaku-e*[13], and the point 3 cm in front of *Hyaku-e* is called *Zen-chō*[14], and the point 3 cm behind *Hyaku-e* is called *Go-chō*[15]. Press these front and back points, namely *Zen-chō* and *Go-chō,* with your fingers. In addition, press the left and right sides of the head. Next, press the forehead. Then you will feel refreshed.

When you are absent-minded, your shoulders, back, the back of your neck and so on are stiff and blood flow in your brain is in a congested state. If you apply acupressure to these areas to improve the blood flow, the function of your brain will become more active. If you apply this simple treatment and then start working or studying, you will engage more efficiently.

(5) How to relieve insomnia
Some people complain that they suffer from insomnia, but there is no such thing as insomnia. Due to incomplete, shallow sleep, they cannot get a good night's sleep and so they feel as if they didn't sleep much. In this case, the length of sleep does not matter.

Even if you only sleep for three or four hours, if you sleep soundly, you will not lack sleep. But in the long run, sleep of seven or eight hours a night is reasonable. Even Napoleon would not have always slept for a short time.

Insomnia which comes with lack of sound sleep occurs where the parasympathetic nervous system, which takes the lead when sleeping, and the sympathetic nervous system, which takes the lead when awake, do not alternate in a good rhythm, and both nervous systems work imperfectly.

---

[13] An important acupoint. The word means the point where a hundred (many) meridians meet.
[14] This word means the front top.
[15] This word means the back top.

In terms of the physical body, people with insomnia cannot relax their whole body. Particularly they cannot relax the lower back, and the chest muscles are tight, which makes them unable to breathe comfortably.

Not only people with insomnia but also those whose minds are tense have muscle contraction in the shoulders, neck and chest and find it hard to sleep. Also, if you have an abnormality in your stomach, heart, or liver, you may not be able to sleep or may sleep too much.

Therefore, in order to fall asleep smoothly, it is advisable to take light exercise or a warm bath in order to relax the whole body and also spend some time to relax your mind, for example, watching a fun television program.

Eating before going to sleep will eventually raise your body temperature and interfere with a good night's sleep.

(6) How to relieve toothache

Tooth decay is caused by bacteria, and so even if you massage the area, there will be no effect. For other toothaches, acupressure, massage, moxibustion and so on will be effective. When you have toothache due to overwork or a cold, your shoulders and neck are very stiff and your gums have blood congestion.

In this case, first massage the neck and shoulders by pressing with your fingers or grabbing with your hands. Next, massage in a twisting motion the area between your lower chin and temples with your index, middle and ring fingers. Furthermore, you can apply acupressure to the painful area.

(7) How to correct physical distortion in daily life

Look at the right shoulder of a barber who is cutting somebody's hair with scissors in his right hand from morning till evening all day long. You can see that his right shoulder is raised up.

Look closely at the right shoulder of a dentist who is looking into someone's decayed tooth. You can see that the dentist's right shoulder is lowered down.

This kind of body distortion occurs in daily movements. These must be rebalanced by other movements or exercises. Always keep in mind that you must maintain balance.

For example:

① If your right shoulder is lower than the left, hold your luggage under your right arm, or hang it from your left hand. (Do the reverse on the other side.)

② When walking, increase the stride length of the shorter leg.

③ When running on a round course, run with the shorter leg on the outer side of the circle.

④ When cleaning with a cloth in your hand, do it with your weaker hand.

⑤ When using a vacuum cleaner, you should hold the suction pipe in the opposite way to your usual habit as you put one hand away from your body and the other near to it. The position of your feet will change accordingly. The way the body twists depends on which side of the body the equipment is placed.

⑥ When squeezing a rag, the influence on the body depends on which hand moves away from your body. You should practise the way that feels difficult.

⑦ The way your body twists depends on whether the bookshelf in the office is on your right side or left. The arrangement of chairs and desks is also important. It is a good point to rearrange them sometimes in order not to create distortion of the body.

⑧ Normal daily movements are easily done subconsciously. So, you tend to use only the hands and feet that are easier to use, for example, when lifting something onto a shelf, climbing stairs, picking something up, putting on your shoes, taking off your shoes, and so on. All that you have to do is to consciously act and do the opposite of your normal habit. Using the body distortedly is unavoidable, but the problem is that it becomes fixed.

⑨ However, in any case, if you do the opposite too much, you will get a new distortion, so be sure to check your body carefully so that you do not overdo it.

Ⅲ

Yoga during Your Commute

- How to enjoy a crowded train

Morning exercises to start the day comfortably

In order to wake up comfortably in the morning and start the day, a good night's sleep is necessary. This is because a good night's sleep relieves the fatigue from the previous day and replenishes your energy. If you stay up all night for work or fun, you will remain tired and your energy will not be replenished. So, your body will be more tired than you can imagine. Even if you feel good by having finished off your work, that feeling is only temporary, and the tiredness will surface later.

Ideally, you should wake up feeling refreshed with the willingness to move into immediate action arising from within. On the contrary, if your body is heavy with your head dull and unclear and you still want to sleep, this is proof that your body has an abnormality somewhere or is tired so that new energy is not being generated. It is an unhealthy awakening.

A good night's sleep is required for getting rid of an abnormal awakening, but the problem is not always a lack of sleep. If you wake up once but then go back to sleep again and again because you are still sleepy, your autonomic nerves will be disturbed, which does not lead to a good physical condition. The transition from sleep to awakening is the transition from a phase led by the parasympathetic nerves to a phase led by the sympathetic nerves. So, we must devise a way to ease this transition.

In yoga, the following activities are carried out to start the day comfortably. We call these 'morning practice'.

First, we do a warm-up and corrective exercise called 'Sun Salutation' (Fig.17).

This exercise is based on movements for worshiping the sun or a deity at a temple. Its purpose is to correct the body's left-right imbalance, stretch the muscles that tend to contract (such as the muscles of the back of the legs), and bend forwards and

Fig.17 Sun Salutation

1 Stand upright. Put your palms together with your middle fingers at eye level and elbows stretched sideways but not higher than shoulder level

2 With your palms together, extend your arms upwards. If your feet are slightly apart and big toes are strong, you will feel strength around your abdomen and hips

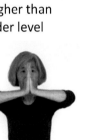

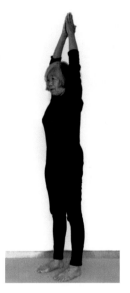

3 While exhaling, bend forwards and downwards. Catch your ankles and pull your abdomen in

4 (right) Put your hands on the floor. Pull your right foot backwards

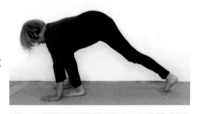

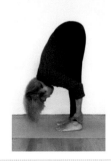

5 (right) While inhaling, raise your upper body and look up

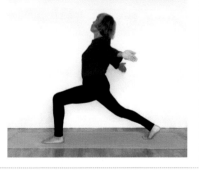

6 While exhaling, bring your hands back to the floor at both sides of your left foot, pull your left foot backwards next to the right foot, and raise your hips high to create a peaklike form

7 While inhaling, bring your right foot forwards, raise your upper body and look up

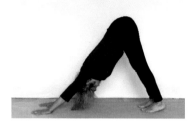

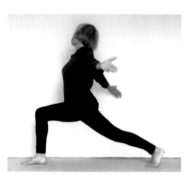

8 While exhaling, repeat Step 6 with the opposite feet

9 While inhaling, lower your chest to the floor, then lower your hips to the floor and bend your torso backwards

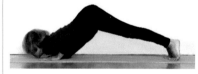

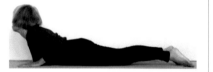

10 While exhaling, lower your torso and rest your forehead on the floor. Regulate your breathing

11 While inhaling bit by bit, slowly and deeply, raise your head and then ribcage as if moving one vertebra at a time. Bend your torso backwards

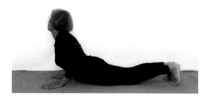

12 Hold your breath, lower your chest and raise your hips. While exhaling, create a peaklike form

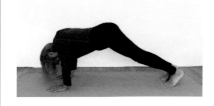 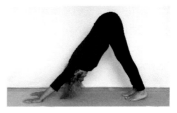

13 Repeat Step 7 and Step 8

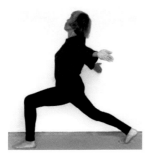

14 (left) While inhaling, bring your left foot forwards, raise your upper body. Look up

15 (right) While exhaling, bring your right foot forwards next to your left foot

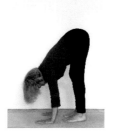

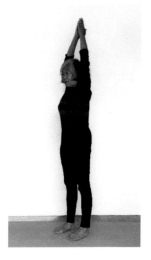

16 (left) While inhaling, put your palms together and then straighten up your body as in Step 2

17 (right) While exhaling, bring your hands in front as in Step 1

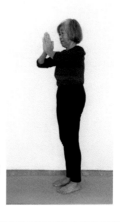

backwards repeatedly to make the spine flexible. By carrying out this exercise, both sides of the ribcage become balanced, and the autonomic nerves become stable.

After this exercise, we take a cold shower or bath. If we take a warm bath in the morning, our body will become too loose and our mind will become unfocused. So, by stimulating the sympathetic nerves with cold water, we encourage a smooth transition from the sleeping state, which is dominated by the parasympathetic nerves.

The principles of training in my yoga *dōjō* are to alternate opposing stimuli such as static and dynamic, warm and cold, slow and intense, mental and physical, in order to not be one-sided. This is because such alternating stimuli help to create balance in our mind and body and ease the transition between the activation of the parasympathetic and sympathetic nervous systems.

Purification exercises help your excretion

While you sleep at night, you recover from tiredness, store new energy and also prepare for eliminating toxins and unnecessary substances. You must support these functions so that they work smoothly.

The following are toxins and unnecessary substances which are harmful if kept in the body:

(1) Gas: residual gas in the lungs and intestines
(2) Fluid: urine and sweat
(3) Solid: faeces
(4) Overall: residual energy and so on.

In order to eliminate these, we in yoga perform 'purification exercises', which promote defecation, urination and gas removal.

The features of these exercises are as follows:

(1) To replace residual gas in the lungs with fresh air by moving the diaphragm vertically and opening and closing the ribcage.

(2) To promote blood circulation throughout the body, activate intestinal peristalsis, raise body temperature, sweat, and enhance kidney function, by active movements of stretching, contracting and twisting, while focusing on the waist and abdomen.

(3) To consume residual energy, by giving out as much energy as possible.

Now, I will explain how to perform these purification exercises. Please also refer to Fig.18.

① Stand with your legs wide apart, interlace your fingers with your palms facing outwards, and extend your arms forwards, parallel to the floor. Next, with your back straight, twist your upper body and neck to the left while exhaling, bringing the arms to the left at the same time as if you are drawing a semi-circle with them. Then, do the reverse for the right side.

② Open both legs wide and stretch your Achilles tendons with your toes turned slightly inwards. Place your hands on the floor in front of you. Your fingers are spread apart. While inhaling, raise your hips and stretch your spine. While keeping your hips as they are, bend your arms, and stick out your chin. Then while exhaling, bring your upper body forwards. When you reach a position you cannot hold any longer, drop your hips suddenly, arch your upper body backwards, and raise your chin upwards. Repeat this about 30 times.

③ Open both legs wide, place your hands shoulder-width apart on the floor, straighten your arms and lower your hips down.

While exhaling, twist your upper body and neck to the right to look at your left heel. At the same time, turn both heels to the left. Then do the reverse for the other side. Repeat these about 30 times.

Fig.18 Purification exercises

① Twisting your abdomen, hips and back promotes blood circulation in the abdominal area. This helps to remove inflammation, blood congestion and adhesions

② This exercise activates the function of the nerves and hormones

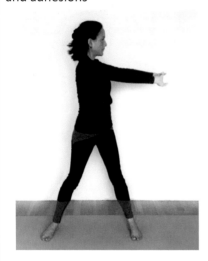

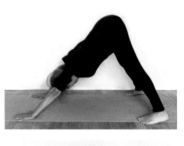

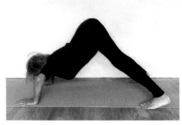

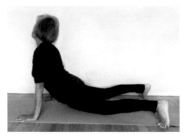

③ Repeatedly twisting your wrists, ankles and lower back activates the function of your intestines, thus improving bowel movement

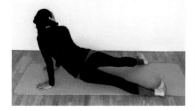 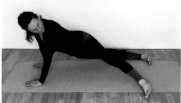

④ This exercise alternately heightens your abdominal pressure and chest pressure and activates the function of your autonomic nervous system. Breathing practices increase your excretion power

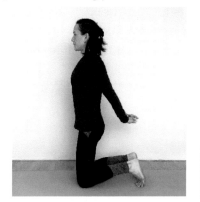 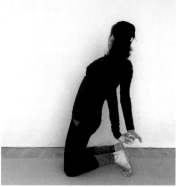

④ Kneel down with your knees hip-width apart and interlace your fingers behind your body with palms facing outwards. While inhaling, raise your arms with your wrists twisted further. While exhaling, slowly arch your body backwards from the knees. Push your abdomen forwards and bend backwards until your hands touch your left heel. Keeping this position, pull your chin in and gaze forwards. Come back up to a straight position. Do this again, but this time touching your right heel. Repeat this several times.

Breakfast as taught by yoga

Recently, increasing numbers of people seem to skip breakfast. It is not uncommon for children to miss this meal too. However, it is generally said that breakfast should not be skipped. Is this true?

I don't think there is any data yet showing that people who skip breakfast have a short life. In yoga, the meal pattern of a day is taught as follows:

According to the rhythm of the life force, morning is the time for excretion. If we eat too much, blood will collect in our stomach, which will not help excretion. Therefore, it is taught that lunch is the main meal to replenish nutrition.

Some people skip breakfast, eat a simple lunch, and eat a big supper. This is unnatural from the above-mentioned perspective. Because the principle of diet is to 'use what is put in', we should eat breakfast just to supply nutrition until lunch time. And it is better to have a bigger nutritious lunch and a simple supper.

As for the content of food, it is better to eat mainly alkaline food in the morning because the body acidifies during the daytime. In my yoga *dōjō, we take only miso[16] soup with a lot of vegetables for breakfast. The action of the enzymes in the miso enhances nutritious power. Also, when a small amount of food enters the stomach, the peristaltic movement of the intestines is promoted for better excretion.

Habits are created, even with meals. So, if you skip breakfast, your body will adapt to that, and if you take breakfast, you will become unable to miss it.

---

[16] A traditional fermented soybean-based paste used in Japanese cuisine.

The faster you walk to the station, the better for your body

I have already mentioned that a good night's sleep is important for a good awakening. I have also introduced cold bathing and morning exercises. However, the quickest way to wake up from drowsiness is to walk fast. For commuting to work or school by train, it is good to walk from home to the station, and from the other station to the office or school. You can also jog.

Let's consider our feet, based on what yoga teaches. For human beings to become able to stand on two feet, it is said that the first prerequisite was that the first toes (big toes) became particularly developed. This sounds convincing when compared to the feet of a monkey.

When the first toes are well developed like a human's and the gaps between the first and second toes are small, it is easier to apply force to the sole of the foot. Yogic training methods for the feet include standing on one leg, skipping, wearing iron clogs, wearing Japanese wooden one-tooth *geta* sandals, running on a slope or sand, and walking on a tightrope. The common purpose of these methods is to develop the first toes.

The strength of the big toes very much relates to standing or walking. In the correct standing posture, the weight of the upper body directly falls to the arches of the feet. Strong big toes make the Achilles tendons strong, which makes it easier to support body weight.

Compared to this, the feet of a monkey have strength in the fifth toes, which creates a forward-leaning posture that looks very unstable to support the weight of their upper body.

In other words, if we take a forward-leaning posture with the weight more supported by the fifth toes and heels, we might give the unavoidable resemblance of a monkey's figure. I call this 'a posture of fatigue'.

I must say that this posture would bring us difficulty in leading a human life and enhancing intelligence. As evidence, we are in this monkey-like posture whenever we are dominated by instinctive desires or animal-like emotions.

Please never stand like a monkey. When walking, put strength into your big toes. These toes also help to determine the direction in which you walk.

Now I will explain how to walk in crowded places when commuting to work or school. Please take a good standing posture, as already explained, with your chest open, strength put into your lower back, your chin pulled in and the back of your neck stretched. Then, try to move forwards from your hips, not just from your legs.

When you are about to bump into someone, twist your body from your lower back and bring either shoulder forwards in front of you to avoid the collision or to slip through the crowd. At this time, the big toes take an important role.

It is good if both big toes have power. If one foot has strength in its heel and the other foot has strength in its big toe, the position of the spine tends to be distorted, which could cause hemorrhoids or menstrual pain. Also, if your feet are not strong, your upper body will try to protect them, which makes it hard for you to relax.

By looking at the soles of your shoes, you can see where the centre of gravity of your body falls.

If it falls to the arches of the feet, the soles of your shoes will be worn evenly. This is evidence that your feet and lower body have been trained to be well balanced. If your feet are turned rightwards (or leftwards), make the right (or left) foot take a wider stride than the other.

How to endure being pushed in a crowded train

When the departure bell rings and you think no more people will come into the carriage, suddenly many people push inside. At this time, people standing by the opposite door receive great pressure.

Even so, while heading to your office, you might feel slightly superior to those who missed the train.

If the train journey time is short, it will not be too bad. But the commuting distance of office workers is getting longer year by year. If you must experience this every day, it will be wise for everyday life to know how to spend your time in a crowded train.

What can you do when you are pushed inside by force and almost crushed? It is the same as walking. Put strength into your big toes, pull your chin in, stretch the back of your neck, tighten your anal muscles, and keep your strength in the *tanden*. And make sure that no unnecessary force is applied to other areas. Think of yourself as a willow tree. The willow is flexible but has a strong core. It can withstand external pressure. So, instead of pushing back when you are pushed, relax your shoulders and let your '*ki*' pass straight through to the other side.

'*Ki*' is also called *prāna*. It is vital energy, the life force itself. Also, this has positive and negative qualities. Utilise these and make your morning rush hour fun without wasting your energy.

In order to pass your *ki* through, you need to relax your muscles with a smile and imagine that you are being pulled towards a wall or window in the opposite direction, instead of pushing back the person who is pushing you. By doing this, you can create a state as if you are resisting, without actually exerting a force of resistance. Remember that, when you hit a drum, the vibrations are also transmitted to the other side which the drumstick does not touch.

Yogic training in a crowded train

(1) <u>Standing on your big toes</u> (Fig.19)
You can continue physical training even on the train or bus while commuting to work or school. I will first explain a method of standing on your big toes. If you stand on your big toes, your *tanden*'s power will be strengthened.

In this training, open your feet hip-width apart, raise your heels to stand on your big toes, and finally shift your weight from the little toe side to the big toe side. There, support your weight mainly on the big toes for 8 to 10 seconds. Rest and repeat.

(2) <u>Grabbing the hanging straps</u> (Fig.20)
Normally, the hanging straps in a train are there only to prevent you from falling over. However, you can use them for training to stimulate and strengthen your internal organs, fingers, brain and so on.

For example, hold one of the hanging straps firmly with your five fingers and then loosen your hold. Repeat these actions. The five fingers are closely related to the lower back and cerebrum. So, this training is characterised by the strengthening effect on these parts.

Its effectiveness depends on how you breathe and use your conscious mind. I will add some important points as follows:

When grabbing the strap tightly, hold the entire strap while exhaling and pulling your abdomen in, and be aware that you are grabbing it with abdominal strength. Don't think that you are holding it with your fingers.

By doing this, your whole body cooperates with your hand which holds the strap, and this becomes a stimulus to strengthen the body. If you keep your focus on the hand, only the hand will get tired.

If your posture is hunched forwards, hold a strap in each hand and arch the body backwards.

If your shoulders are uneven, hold the strap with the hand on the side of the lower shoulder.

If your body is twisted, adjust the position of your shoulders, hips and legs so that your body twists in the opposite direction.

Fig.19 Standing on your big toes	Fig.20 Grabbing the hanging straps	Fig.21 Heel breathing
Stay in this position for 8 to 10 seconds. Rest and repeat	Grab the strap with abdominal strength	Raise your heels while inhaling, and hold your breath when your heels are raised fully

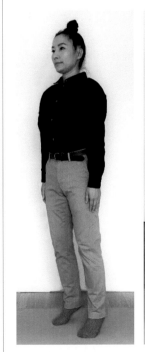 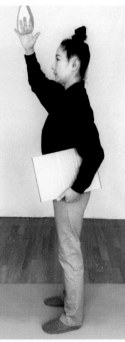 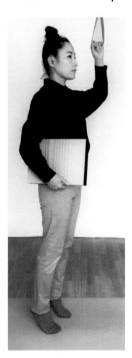

(3) Heel breathing (Fig.21)

This is similar to the method of standing on your big toes, which was mentioned earlier, but here the emphasis is on breathing.

While you keep your hand on the strap in the train, straighten your spine and put your feet together. Raise your heels while inhaling and hold your breath when your heels are raised fully (for about 3-5 seconds at first, then gradually increasing the time). When you feel it is enough, slowly lower your heels to the floor while exhaling little by little. Although this is a simple method, moving your heels up and down is an exercise for your whole body, which stimulates and activates all the muscles of the body.

Another method is to raise your heels and drop them back down with a thud, which is effective for relaxing the whole body, stimulating the soles of the feet and awakening the brain. In Chinese medicine, this exercise is said 'to eliminate a hundred diseases'.

(4) One-legged standing (Fig.22)

If you stand on one leg, you will naturally feel the strength gathering in the *tanden.* It also straightens your spine, tightens your anal muscles, and increases your ability to maintain balance. It is also effective for people with hemorrhoids.

One-legged standing can be done as follows: when standing on your right leg, put the instep of your left foot against the calf of your right leg. When you get tired, change legs. Standing on the right leg is good for your stomach, and standing on the left leg is good for your liver. It is okay for you to do this only for a short time.

A general physical fitness test may also ask you to stand on one leg with your eyes closed. If you wobble immediately, it is a sign that your body is aging.

Fig.22 One-legged standing	Fig.23 Standing meditation on the train	Fig.24 Sitting meditation on the train
Standing on your right leg is good for your stomach. Standing on your left leg is good for your liver	Slowly take a deep abdominal breath through your nose	Sit in a good posture. Breathe deeply

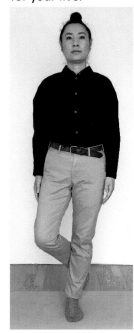 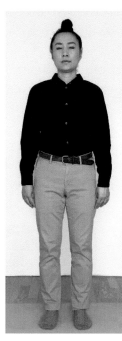 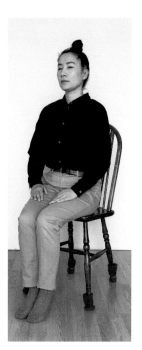

(5) <u>Standing meditation on the train</u> (Fig.23)
Open your feet body-width apart and straighten your back and the back of your neck. Pull your chin in a little, stretch your chest, and relax your shoulders. Turn your knees slightly inwards and pull your buttocks backwards so that your weight falls to the arches of the feet. Then, close your eyes lightly and slowly take a

deep abdominal breath through your nose. Put strength into your big toes and maintain balance with your knees and hips.

(6) <u>Sitting meditation on the train</u> (Fig.24)
Pull your hips deeply to the back of the seat, then as if pushing your waist forwards, open your chest with your shoulders and neck relaxed. Create a state in which your anal muscles are firm and lower abdomen has strength. Pull your chin in and extend the back of your neck as if the top of your head is pointing towards heaven.

Then, put your hands on your waist, lift your knees slightly, and while keeping the knees naturally open, bring your feet back to the floor. Put strength into the inner sides of your knees and big toes. Hold a *mudrā*[17] and lightly place your hands on your thighs. Then maintain this good posture and breathe deeply. (It is best to maintain a posture in which the lower legs are perpendicular to the floor).

Exercises to recover from tiredness while waiting for the train

(1) <u>How to alleviate shoulder stiffness while standing</u>
Straighten your back and open your chest. Raise both shoulders together fully while inhaling and hold the tension for a few seconds. Then suddenly release it. If you repeat this a few times, your shoulders will be lighter with the stiffness loosened.

(2) <u>How to alleviate back pain while standing</u>
Stand with your feet slightly apart, place your hands on your waist and rotate your hips slowly, making big circles. Rotate

---

[17] A *mudrā* is a symbolic or ritual hand gesture or bodily pose used in yoga-based spiritual practice.

clockwise and counterclockwise, three times each way. Still keeping your hands on your waist, gently twist your upper body to the right while exhaling. Then twist to the left. Do this three times in each direction. It is also good to push your waist rightwards and leftwards.

(3) How to lift drooping internal organs

With both hands on your lower abdomen, exhale fully while pulling your abdomen in completely. Next, without inhaling through your nose or mouth, spread your ribs as if you were inhaling, and stretch your chest. This action makes entire internal organs get sucked upwards. Repeat this several times.

(4) How a person who overeats can correct their posture by holding a bag

People who overeat are generally bent forwards and have their right shoulder raised. Correcting the stooped posture and levelling both shoulders will help to change their overeating tendency.

Hold a bag in your left hand, which makes the left shoulder go up and the right shoulder go down. And open the chest. This effort will help to correct the raised right shoulder as well as the stooped posture.

You can also improve the condition of your eyes yourself

People are worried that their legs will become weak, and so try to walk or run. People whose stomach or intestines are weak try to strengthen these organs in various ways. However, if their eyesight becomes weak, people tend to accept it as unavoidable heredity and start using glasses. There is a widespread belief that abnormal eyesight is irreversible, but this is incorrect. In order to have healthy eyes, your mind and body must first be healthy.

Here, I will show you acupressure methods to improve the condition of your eyes, which you can easily do on the way to work or school. First, close your eyes and apply acupressure to the area around your eyes and temples. In addition, it is good for your eyes if you rotate your wrists, extend and twist your arms, and turn your face upwards and relax. This is because, when your hands, shoulders and neck are tense, the blood in your eyes becomes congested and, as a result, they tire easily.

Rub your palms and cover your eyes with cupped hands without giving pressure to the eyeballs. This will improve blood circulation in your eyes.

If the sun is shining, lightly close your eyes while leaning towards the window, or blink your eyes to stimulate the lacrimal glands and relieve the tension. In soft sunlight, open your eyes and bathe them in the sunlight.

The easiest exercise you can do on the train is as follows: gaze at something far away and then look at something close by to stretch and contract the muscles around the eyes.

A well-known nutritionist, who investigates the ecology of African animals based on their food and the dietary habits of indigenous peoples, said, "There are many vigorous indigenous people over 80 years old. Jungle life in Africa is monotonous, but very few people in this area have been seen wearing glasses." According to this nutritionist, it is because they look at the far horizon on the African continent. Of course, they have no televisions, newspapers or magazines.

Next, let's try applying acupressure to six sets of acupoints for the eyes, which can be easily done even on the train. If you do this, perhaps you won't have to go to Africa to look at the horizon for your eye exercises.

The first set of points is below the earlobes, behind the jaw. Press the points on both sides with your thumbs, up towards your eyes. Also rub and squeeze them.

The second set of points is in the middle of the sterno-cleidomastoid muscles, which run diagonally from under the

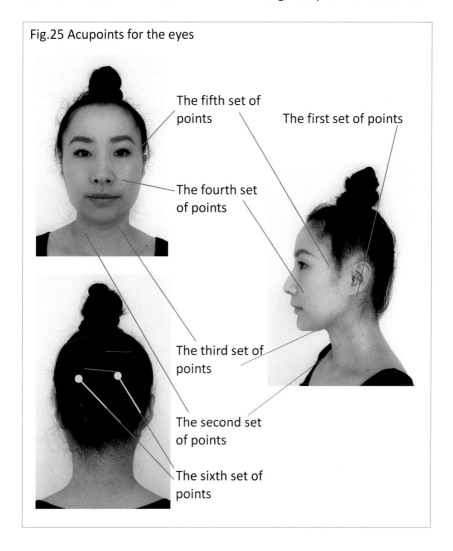

Fig.25 Acupoints for the eyes

The fifth set of points

The first set of points

The fourth set of points

The third set of points

The second set of points

The sixth set of points

ears to the lowest part of the throat. Press the points on both sides with your index fingers, as if you are poking them inwards.

The third set of points is under the lower jaws, diagonally upwards from the Adam's apple. Press the points on both sides with your index fingers, as if you are pushing them towards the eyes, and rub them with pressure.

The fourth set of points is beside the nose wings, below the cheekbones. Apply acupressure to the points on both sides, as if you are lifting them towards the eyes with the index fingers.

The fifth set of points is at the depression of the temples. Apply acupressure to the points on both sides with your thumbs while supporting the back of your head with the other fingers. Rub and squeeze the points as well.

To find the sixth set of points, draw an imaginary, horizontal line from the top of the ears to the back of the head, and find a very shallow hollow just behind each eye. Apply acupressure to the points on both sides, pressing them towards the direction of the eyes with your thumbs.

A self-diagnosis method that you can use on the train

It may come as a surprise to some people that the hand represents the internal organs. The entire hand is related to the brain. Please touch and feel your hands which are under continuous tension every day. Are your hands tight? If so, you have accumulated tiredness.

Anyway, tiredness of the brain correlates with tiredness of the hands. So, when your brain feels tired, exercise your hands to relieve tension. You should use your hands in a relaxed state. When your hands are tense, your brain becomes excited.

Now, I will explain about the relationship between each part of the hand and the internal organs. By looking at someone's hands, you could tell the condition of that person's internal organs at a glance. You can make a self-diagnosis based on the colour of your hands, the shape of your fingers, and the colour of your nails. You could say your hands are a barometer of your health.

(1) <u>The relationship between the fingers and the internal organs</u>
① Thumb: This is related to the parasympathetic nerves and to keeping the blood alkaline. Rubbing the bulge at the base of the thumb (thenar) stimulates the parasympathetic nerves and calms you down. Also, if you rub the root of your thumb and index finger, it will stimulate the intestines and liver and increase your ability to excrete.
② Index finger: This is related to the liver, stomach, and intestines, which are digestive organs. Overeating makes the index finger stiff. The right index finger relates to the liver and the left relates to the stomach.
③ Middle finger: This is related to the heart, kidneys, and blood vessels. When you feel a sudden abnormality in your heart, it may be calmed by pressing the centre of the palm (an acupoint called *Rōkyū*) just below the middle finger of the left hand. When straightening your hand, if the middle finger bends to the little finger side, you have an alkaline constitution, if the middle finger bends to the thumb side, you have an acidic constitution.
④ Ring finger: This is related to the nervous system including the part of the central nervous system that is connected to vision. That is why someone who has a long ring finger is said to have excellent artistic ability.
⑤ Little finger: This is related to the genital organs and sympathetic nerves. Strengthening your little finger is also directly linked to energy boosting.

Rotate, pull and squeeze each of your fingers. Rotate its every section and rub the palm well. As the blood circulation in your hands improves, you will feel your entire body becoming lighter.

However, you might put too much strength in the hand doing the massage. So, be careful not to stiffen the shoulder on that side. Do these movements while exhaling with your arms relaxed from the shoulders to the fingertips.

(2) How to detect liver fatigue from the fingers

Align the little finger, ring finger, and middle finger straight. When you try to bend the second joint of the index finger horizontally, it bends at a diagonal angle. Then if you force it to bend horizontally, the other fingers may separate. This shows that your liver is weakened.

(3) Self-diagnosis by looking at the palm of your hands

The colour of the palm is closely related to your health: white shows weakness in lungs; black—kidney, purple—circulatory system, blue—gastrointestinal tract, green—spleen, yellow—liver, and red—heart.

(4) Self-diagnosis by looking at your fingernails

Healthy fingernails are pink and glossy. Fingernails that are overly red indicate hyperaemia, hot flushes, fever, or congestion of arterial blood in the fingertips. Pale fingernails indicate anaemia. When there is swelling in your body, your fingernails become whitish.

Bluish fingernails are caused by stagnation of venous blood. When this condition becomes worse, the fingernail colour darkens. This indicates a lack of oxygen in the blood. Yellowish fingernails indicate an abnormality in the liver, and a cloudy white colour throughout is a sign of cirrhosis.

Vertical ridges on the fingernails are common in older people, and also in those who have a weakness in their heart. This indicates abnormality in nutrient metabolism. People who have brittle fingernails are deficient in calcium and prone to catching colds. This is due to excessive intake of white sugar, lack of water, or abnormality in thyroid hormones, and indicates that calcium is dissolving into the blood.

A hangnail at the root of a fingernail is caused by a lack of vitamin C or overeating. Clearly visible lunulae indicate great intestinal absorption. When you have a high fever, a deep horizontal groove would appear on a fingernail. A spoon nail indicates iron deficiency anaemia. If your fingernail is coming off the nail bed, it indicates an abnormality in the thyroid gland.

How to drive a car without getting tired

Driving a car is no longer a special skill. Whether we like it or not, we cannot think of living without a car. As we all know, riding in or driving a car has detrimental effects on the health of our legs and lower back.

However, when we consider that car travel makes our commute easier and diversifies the way we spend our leisure time, there are lots of benefits to it. Here, let's think about ways to drive a car safely without getting tired or giving rise to abnormalities. First, we will look at the posture we take when we drive.

The correct posture for driving is a posture in which your hands and shoulders are relaxed and free. This is because you cannot move freely unless you are relaxed.

You must hold the steering wheel so lightly that you can hardly feel whether you are holding it or not. If your hands are tense, you will not be able to manoeuvre it smoothly, which is dangerous. When your thoughts are elsewhere, it is easy to cause an accident. This is because tension in your brain also makes your hands tense. When the hands and legs are relaxed, the head and neck are also relaxed. That way, you can pay attention to all directions.

In other words, if you don't put extra force into your hands, you can relax your brain, which creates some space for your attention and allows you to manoeuvre the steering wheel freely. To stop thinking, you must relax your hands. Recall that the hands and brain are interconnected.

When your limbs and mind are relaxed and only your abdomen has strength, your intuition works sharply, so that you can turn the steering wheel in the right direction instantly. If you must think and act, it can be too late.

No matter how much you try to devise your own driving posture, it is almost determined by the car seat. If you can adjust the seat forwards, backwards, sideways or vertically, please position the seat where you can relax and have a wide view. Trying to look cool like a racer is a bad idea.

Pull your chin in, relax your shoulders and arms, put your strength in the *tanden*, and relax your legs except the feet which operate the pedals. If you feel tired or nervous, stop the car, raise your feet and rest. Keep your upper body always relaxed. These are the basic keys to the correct driving posture.

Next, how can you avoid accidents? There are three points to consider:

(1) Observe traffic regulations

(2) Being familiar with the geography, that is, being familiar with what you are handling

(3) Pay even and relaxed attention to other vehicles and the situation

I will explain these three points, as follows:

(1) refers to the social order to protect everyone's freedom. If you follow the rules, you will be protected by the rules.

(2) refers to the object you are dealing with. You can be reassured when you know what you are dealing with, and so, accidents due to tension are less likely to occur. You will fear what you don't know. When you do something with a relaxed mind, you will be more able to exert your full power and avoid mistakes.

(3) When you try hard not to fall into a hole, you may actually fall in. The best way to do something is by doing it with the *mu-mind. The *mu-mind is an empty mind, a mind of non-attachment to anything. Therefore, you can pay attention to everything evenly. If you pay attention to other cars and things with the *mu-mind, you will be able to deal with things instantly.

If you get used to driving a car, you will be able to do it with the *mu-mind. In this sense, driving a car has much in common with zazen.

An expert driver pays attention by listening though they don't seem to be listening, and by looking though they don't seem to be looking. This is the only way to be aware of the whole situation: what is happening far and near, left and right, and in front and behind. You cannot drive a car very safely with a single-pointed focus.

Therefore, it is easy to manoeuvre a well-made car smoothly. That is not the case with a car which does not work well.

Now, I will explain some easy exercises you can do before driving, during a break, or when you are tired from driving. Please refer to Fig.26.

Fig.26 Exercises for car commuters

Exercises to do in the morning. Do each exercise three times

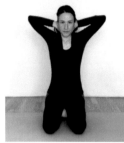 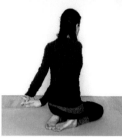 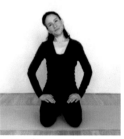

1 Sit in *seiza*. Interlace your fingers behind your neck. Pull your elbows sideways

2 With your fingers interlaced, rotate your arms externally and stretch them

3 Tilt your head back and forth, and side to side

4 Bend your body forwards

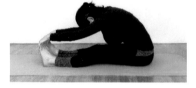

5 Sit in *seiza* and lift your arms. Keeping the same posture, tilt the upper body backwards

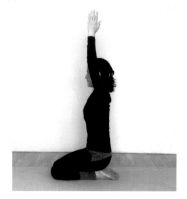 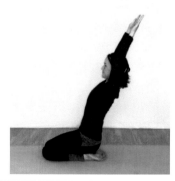

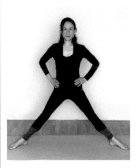

6 (left) Open your legs as widely as you can

7 (right) Stand straight. Then, while lifting the arms in front, bend your legs without raising your heels off the floor

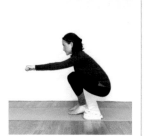

Exercises to do during a break from driving. Do for 30 seconds each

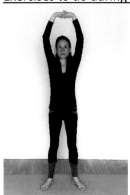

1 (left) Extend your arms upwards. Bend you body side to side

2 (right) Stand straight with your arms around one knee. Try to bring it close to your chest. Do with the other knee as well

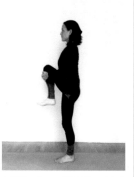

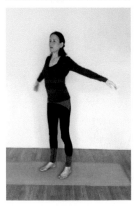

3 (left and right) Swing your arms backwards, upwards and forwards as if drawing a circle. Then cross them in front. Uncross and repeat. It looks like drawing the figure '8'. Bounce up and down, bending your knees throughout.

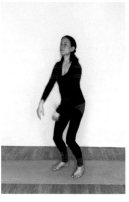

Exercises you can do before going to bed

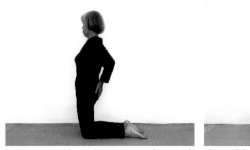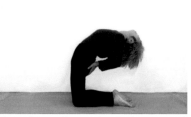

1 Put your hands on your lower back and bend your body backwards

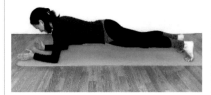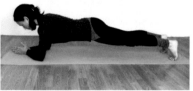

2 Hold your body up with your elbows and toes. Clap your hands together

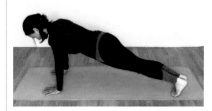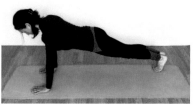

3 In a push-up position, jump to the left and right with both feet together

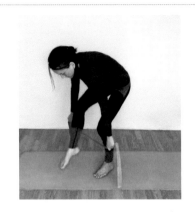

4 Holding a belt in front of you, step over it one leg at a time. Rotate your arms upwards in a semi-circle behind you. Then extend your body and arms upwards. Lower the arms in front to return to the original position

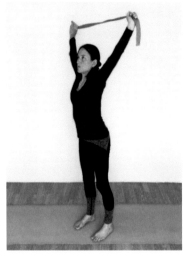

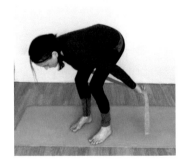

5 Lie on your stomach. Have someone shake your legs gently. Do each leg in turn

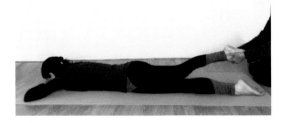

IV

Yoga in the Office

- To have good relationships and improve work efficiency

The yogic way of health through your work

If the work you are doing is someone else's work, it becomes a burden for you. If you don't do your own work, you won't enjoy it.

For example, if you want to ski, you can enjoy it comfortably whether you feel cold or carry heavy equipment. However, it is not very enjoyable if somebody else makes you walk in the cold or carry heavy things when you are not going to ski yourself.

In my yoga *dōjō, I teach students, "Make the work you are involved in your own and do the same with your studies." This way of thinking does not expect a reward or result. If the work or study is so much fun for you, it will lead to your happiness, no matter what. This is a state of good health, mental and physical.

In yoga, a person who thinks that the reward for work is to gain money, or the reward for study is to pass an exam, is called a 'survivor'. This means that they are just living like an animal. Animals wander around in search of food to survive because they have no other choice.

As the English expression 'Enjoy the process' goes, you should set a challenging goal in self-training, self-discipline and self-study, and enjoy studying and working regardless of the result. Without forcing yourself, just keep going in your own way. If you think that you are working for money or studying to pass an exam, it will be a burden for you.

Using a simple example, when you run, you should stop being conscious of other people, as competitive runners do. Instead, if you think that you run for your own health, you will be at ease. It is because you want to compete with others or break a record that running, which should be a healthy sport, becomes harmful. Life is lived every day, and its purpose is not success.

Therefore, in modern times, very few people truly work, from the perspective of yoga. In short, people work because it pays.

In agriculture, whether by using agrochemicals or growing crops out of season, the importance is to grow something that sells... In medical treatment, although it is not good to use medical drugs, it is more profitable to do so ... In manufacturing and commerce as well, profit is the first concern.

You will not be able to achieve joy and a healthy life through work unless you have the realisation that you are doing wonderful work or that you are giving joy to society. A desolate heart may be hidden behind a materially rich lifestyle. Economic growth has made many Japanese people confident in the wrong way. Japan has become an economic power and Japanese people have become like economic animals.

Don't rush! Discover your talents and develop your abilities

You are the person who knows yourself best. So here, I will use myself as an example.

Because I was born as somebody who likes to use their brain, I was never fond of or good at physical activities when I was a child. I practised martial arts since I was little, and I liked it to some extent. However, I was not interested in handicraft or gymnastics, and did not receive good marks for these subjects. I may have looked clumsy and performed poorly to other people, and I myself thought so.

However, there are two cases when somebody is clumsy and unskillful: they are really clumsy and unskillful, or they are so because they are uninterested or unmotivated.

I was judged as poorly skilled at a school that didn't understand my nature, but my parents understood my nature well. They respected my freedom and helped me do whatever I wanted, regardless of whether I was good or poor at it. I was not judged on the surface-level results. So, I didn't feel inferior. Judging somebody as clumsy and unskillful can deny their potential.

Abilities are latent and hidden. They come out in various ways; some people show their talents at an earlier stage in life; others at a later stage. Also, it is possible that, while you are trying something, you gradually become interested in that subject and able to do what you couldn't do before, and that you will become more confident and want to try different things one after another. So, don't judge people as clumsy or poorly skilled, but let them try.

When it comes to school, many parents expect their children to be excellent in all subjects. But when we think about this, it is rather an abnormal state that children are excellent at all subjects. It is unnatural to have no individuality or unique characteristics. Normally everybody has strengths and weaknesses, which is a natural state with individuality and unique characteristics.

We should not deny somebody's weak point but let it be useful. What is often thought to be a weakness often happens to be, in fact, the person's strong point.

In my own case, I am good at thinking, but don't like talking to people. I never dreamt of becoming a person who could make a speech in front of others. However, owing to yoga practice, my weak point has become a strong point. This is due to my practice based on the following teaching learnt from Burmese Sayadaw U Ottama in my childhood, and from Mahatma Gandhi and Master Tempū Nakamura in my youth: Yoga is a learning through experience, in which your own self becomes a teacher as well as student while treating all beings as brothers and sisters. Shakyamuni and Christ also learnt from experience on such a large scale.

To know our own way of life or the way of human life, we should always actively and consciously learn from everything concerning ourselves as I have just explained.

I have experienced more than fifty kinds of professions. I did not work for money, status or honour as people usually do, but for learning. Owing to this wide range of experiences, I was able to grasp principles common among all of them.

To have various stimuli will be an opportunity to develop your talents. You will not understand Japan very well even if you study about it while staying there. To travel around the world and see different parts of it will be a good stimulus for studying about Japan. Whether it is diet or physical training, partial things are harmful and never lead to the development of your abilities. Western athletes seem to practise several types of sport for themselves, thereby enhancing their abilities in their specific sport. In Japan as well, it used to be said, "If you want to master one martial art, you have to do at least 18 types of martial arts (*Bugei Jūhappan*, 武芸十八般)". Certainly, practising as many skills as possible is the basis for developing our abilities and is the way to grasp the truth.

I have so many kinds of work experience: brushing shoes, polishing windows, cleaning, managing a company, teaching at a university, and so on. I think that is why I can explain yoga, which is a philosophy, from the perspective of daily life. Due to these experiences, I can flexibly answer whatever kind of question I receive from anybody.

Ability emerges once you are put in an extreme situation. Trying to figure out what you are good at or what suits you will not lead to answers. Only when being chased by a wolf does your true ability come out. Many people cannot discover themselves because they live a very easy life.

You must not be obsessed with your likes and dislikes. If you are too concerned about the advantages and disadvantages of the things you do, you cannot discover yourself or bring out your abilities fully. If you do not act as if it is a last-ditch attempt, or act with the *mu*-mind, your abilities will not come out. There are many people who usually look incompetent but exert great power when placed in extreme situations.

Also, when somebody can express their ability, it is because there is a need for their ability in that current time and environment. You do not know how much their ability will be assessed in a different time or environment. In the same way, those whose abilities are not regarded very highly may be able to express their skills wonderfully in a time and environment more suited to them. In yoga, it is said that we should have a view of 1000 or 2000 years ahead. Living faithfully to yourself is to develop yourself and to feel the joy of living.

I am not necessarily saying that changing jobs is a good thing. Even for people who must continue the same job, there are an infinite number of ways that things can be thought of or done. They can change their way of thinking or doing things. Discovering what you yourself can do in each situation in your job is to develop your abilities. Only when you realise that will your job become your own work. In yoga, this state in which your work and yourself are united as one is called *sanmai*[18]. Only when you are in this state of *sanmai* will you be able to enjoy your job, which then becomes your work and your way of health.

Boss Type, Obedient Type, Cooperative Type

Whether it is about work or studies, a lot of explanation is needed for some people, and a word is enough for others; some people are quick, and others need more time. Some people can work alone, and others need detailed instructions at all stages. These individual differences are probably innate.

---

[18] Refer to *Samādhi* in Page 178-179 (Chapter 6).

In general, I call people who can work alone the Boss Type, people who need detailed instructions at all stages the Obedient Type, and people who can do with some little instructions the Cooperative Type. You need a good combination of these types of people in your work team.

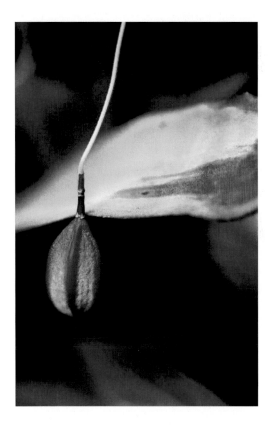

Good combinations are key
when different people work together

When you can't get on with someone

In reality there can be some unpleasant superiors and colleagues at work. What should you do in such a case?

First of all, before you say that somebody is unpleasant, please reflect on whether you understand that person well. Some good points can always be found in people when you get to know them. No one is without merit. We cannot allow ourselves to dislike somebody completely because we all have the value of existence.

Another thing is that there is no one who is completely compatible with you. You like yourself most. There will always be some resistance to something different from you. In other words, it is quite natural that other people are disagreeable, because you are the only one with whom you are compatible.

So, before disliking someone, please think again about the above two points.

Also, always keep in mind that the basis of human relationships is to respect the other person. This is done by having an interest in that person. You can just say, "I appreciate your ongoing support" or "You are brilliant today", and so on. This is the key to good human relationships.

Yoga to improve work efficiency

First of all, you need to be able to concentrate on your work. No special abilities are needed to do that. It is possible if the conditions for concentration are met. They can be summarised by the following three points:

(1) You know the work
(2) You are interested in the work
(3) You need to do the work (you have a purpose).

If these conditions are met, you or anybody should be able to concentrate on the work. I will explain these three points:

(1) If you don't know the content of the work and how to accomplish it, you cannot engage yourself in it. If you must work without knowing what it is, you will be anxious and inefficient. Therefore, when asking someone to do some work, they will not be motivated if you ask them to obediently do what you instruct. They will be much more motivated if you explain the reason and necessary steps.

(2) Interest. This is obvious. However, I can add the following: We are not interested in everything from the start. So, for yourself to be interested in something, you must not have a prejudice without trying it. Furthermore, to attract other people's interest, you must show them enough material so that they feel convinced. If you think only about your own convenience but not of others, you will not succeed even if you can attract their interest. If you want to have their attention and get them to continue working, you need to clearly show them the bigger picture relating to the work.

(3) Purpose. Humans can calculate, unlike animals. Work cannot be done without the prospect of meaning, significance, effect and outcome. Nowadays, even if you just say, "Let's do our best", nobody will do their best. People cannot do that if they don't understand the reason.

Even if you say, "Run", you cannot make people run. However, if you explain the benefits of running repeatedly, the number of runners will grow. Meanwhile, some of them may forget about such benefits and become interested in just running. Anyway, people need to have a sense of value when they are engaged in something.

Tips for not failing at work

The mindset when starting work is *mushin*, the *mu*-mind. The *mu*-mind means unconditional mind, or the mind of non-attachment.

It is courageous to have the determination to do something no matter what may happen. But this is wrong. Don't be heroic and say, "I must do it" or "I have decided I should do it". Unknowingly, this becomes a burden in your mind and disturbs its flexible activity. 'Do with the *mu*-mind' means 'Just do without pretentiousness'. You should just focus on what you do. This is also called 'one mind'.

A certain condition is needed to work with the *mu*-mind. It is daily preparation. Because you don't know well what you are doing, your mind becomes stiff, saying, "I must do". If you organise and maintain the necessary information and abilities on a regular basis, you will be able to work with the *mu*-mind.

It is too late to lock the barn door after the horse has been stolen. You should always visualise the required state even when not needed and be prepared by practising for the worst case. This is called 'training' or 'discipline' in yoga. Speaking in computer language, training or discipline means to programme yourself in preparation for possible emergencies.

Simply put, familiarise yourself as much as possible with what is relevant to your work.

When you are driving a car and know only one road, you will be troubled once something happens on that road. Also, when you don't know the way to a place you have never visited, you will be too busy looking around to drive safely.

It is no exaggeration to say that this is the difference between those who work well and those who work poorly.

How to think when you are between opposing opinions

It often happens that, though you understand two opposing opinions, you cannot agree with just one of them. It is natural that different people think, feel and act differently about the same thing, although sometimes they agree. In yoga, we always affirm the opinions of others. We deny nothing.

Also, when you are talking with someone, you may find your opinion different from theirs. It is fine to be different. On the other hand, it is fine to be the same. That is natural because everybody is different with different experiences. It is impossible to think that you should have the same opinion as others.

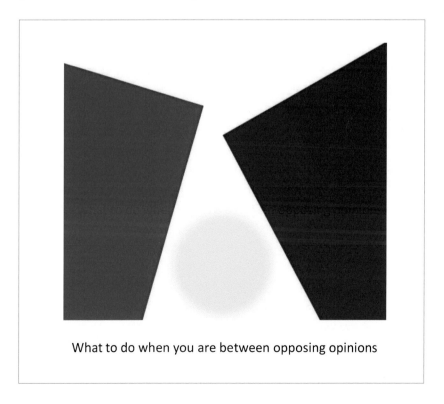

What to do when you are between opposing opinions

Therefore, in the yogic way, we first affirm the other person's opinion even if we want to disagree with it. Affirmation means to accept that there is such a way of thinking. Certainly, there is. That is why they say so. They can only think that way. It is strange to complain, deny, rebel, or get angry against it.

You should say sincerely and respectfully, "Your opinion is a possible way of thinking. If I had your position and experience, I would have thought in the same way as you do. However, because I think from my own position and experience, my opinion is different from yours. So, when we agree with each other, let's work together. I cannot agree with your opinion in this situation. However, it is due to the current situation. If things change, I will adopt your opinion." Like this, you should have an attitude of acknowledging and respecting other people.

It is the same when you are in the middle of different opinions. If two opinions are different, you should express to both sides, "There are different ways of thinking. I understand you both. However, I would think like this." Then you can present your opinion. In this way, the yogic attitude does not deny anything but affirms everything.

When you force someone to follow your way, you are violating them. Taking the perspective I have explained above, you can stand by the truth or the situation rather than side with a particular person.

"I am not against either Mr. A or Mr. B as people. However, when I am asked for my opinion in the current situation, I think I will do what Mr. A says. I am just agreeing with Mr. A's opinion in this case." You had better take this kind of attitude.

None of us humans like to be denied as a person. However, we can cultivate our mind to think as follows: one's opinion does not always need to be agreed with. When there is disagreement, it means one is learning a different way of thinking. So, one can be grateful for that. If everybody thinks like this, quarrels will not be needed.

To utilise everything is the yogic way of thinking.

Two keys to increasing your powers of persuasion

Persuasiveness does not depend on whether you speak nicely or not. Other people listen to you when you speak of what you truly understand or what you have experienced. It is impossible to make others understand what you yourself don't understand well. On the other hand, when you speak from experience, which is your reality, what you say naturally has power.

Please note the following two points:

The opposite of understanding is to not understand. It is also persuasive to say, "I don't understand this." I mean that it is more persuasive to express clearly that you don't understand something instead of pretending to understand it. It is fine to just say, "I will look into it."

Furthermore, 'You have experienced something' does not mean 'You have succeeded in something'. It includes unsuccessful experiences as well. We humans, not being God, experience failure now and then. "I did this activity in this way under this condition but overlooked that point. I guess that was the cause of my failure. So, please be careful when you attempt it" —talking like this will be fine. Our work is done as a new activity based on successes and failures of older generations. It is not only a successful story or good result that has persuasive power.

The other notable point is that, as a proverb says, you should 'adapt your speech to your audience'. However useful your story is, there will be no meaning if it is not understood by the listener. Because you are speaking for the benefit of that person, you must use words they understand and communicate to reach their *mind-heart. Also, a commanding tone works better for some people, and an asking-for-a-favour tone works for others. It depends on what type of person they are, such as a Boss Type or Obedient Type.

The yogic idea to progress a meeting smoothly

There is a key to this, which is different from the aforementioned way where you are between opposing opinions or are facing an opposing opinion.

If you are the facilitator or moderator of the meeting, get someone who is likely to disagree with the agenda to speak first. The moderator should speak as little as possible. This is because people who disagree with the agenda will gradually strengthen their stance if they start by hearing only pro-agenda opinions, and they will have more of a chance to find weakness in those opinions.

You, as the moderator, had better agree with each individual opinion. "I see, I see" will work well. As for opinions that you cannot agree with on the spot, the key is to say, "I cannot agree due to such and such a reason, but if the situation changes, I will be able to agree".

The yogic way is to affirm every opinion. Whether you put it into practice or not is an issue of another dimension.

If you apply what yoga teaches as I have just explained, you will experience much fewer conflicts at work.

Advice for those who do a lot of brain work

Your brain will not work well if it doesn't have good blood circulation. So, before you start work, use your lower body (legs, hips) well. To do this, you can climb up the stairs fast or run during your commute. Jogging in the early morning is very beneficial. Wearing a tight headband serves the purpose of improving blood circulation in the head.

To avoid tiring your brain, it is necessary to pay attention to something completely unrelated in the middle of your workday. This is because the momentary diversion of attention can restore the balance of the brain's function. Take a break and stop thinking about work while, for example, having a cigarette or cup of tea, taking a walk, looking out the window or looking at a painting on the wall.

In order to enhance the function of your brain, it is necessary to raise the blood pressure a little, increase the blood sugar level, and enhance the function of the sympathetic nerves. For this, you had better work in a slightly chilly room, sitting properly on a hard chair rather than a soft chair. Also, a rather empty stomach helps more than a full stomach, as you will probably know from experience.

Be aware that, if you work with a full stomach or sit on a soft chair in a warm room, you may feel too relaxed to focus on your work.

Opening your chest, which is a small easy action, will serve to stop your brain slowing down too quickly. Also, if you momentarily tense your hands sometimes, your brain will function more actively. This is because the hands and brain are linked, and is also effective when you feel drowsy. Also, stretching the muscles of your legs and your Achilles tendons stimulates your brain.

Effective exercises for those who work sitting on a chair

If you work sitting down, please keep the following in mind:

To avoid sitting fatigue, please move your body back and forth and sideways around your tailbone. By stretching the Achilles tendons, you can avoid numbness in your feet.

Backache is often caused by distortion from twisting. To ease this problem, please perform exercises by twisting and bending from your waist while sitting on the chair or standing.

If you sometimes press the area just below your ribs, it will give good stimulation to your liver and stomach. Please do this while exhaling.

People who work looking down should sometimes bend backwards. The stimulation differs depending on the way you bend. So, try different ways.

For those who work standing up, the internal organs tend to droop. It is effective to flex and extend the knees, do a headstand or handstand, breathe deeply, and so on.

For people who work sitting on a chair, the following exercises are effective:

① While you are at your desk, press the desk with your elbows strongly.

② Press your left hip down into the chair and then your right hip. Repeat alternately.

③ Imagine that there is a ball between your knees. Try to press this imaginary ball from both sides.

④ Extend the back of your neck as if pushing the ceiling with your head.

⑤ Place your hands below the seat. Pull the seat as if lifting both the seat and your body.

⑥ Hold your own hands behind your knees. While trying to pull your legs with your arms, straighten and stretch your legs.

⑦ Sit with one leg crossed over the other, grab the chair firmly from both sides, and stretch your legs keeping them crossed. Then try to raise the lower leg and lower the upper leg at the same time, as if squeezing your legs together. Do your best until both legs tremble. This can be done at work, or even on the train.

⑧ Spread both hands on your thighs. Push them down with your palms. At the same time, your thighs try to push up your palms.

⑨ Sitting or standing, interlace your fingers in front of your chest as if praying, and try to pull them apart strongly.

⑩ Place one palm on the side of your head. While your hand pushes, resist the force with your head.

⑪ Put both your hands on your forehead. While your hands push, resist the force with your head.

How to use break times

When you work, you must work hard. If you don't rest during your breaks, you cannot work well when you must work. Similarly, if you don't work when you must work, you cannot rest well when you take a rest. The way to rest varies from person to person. So, you have to discover for yourself what your best way to rest is. Some can rest well by exercising a little, and others by taking a walk, by listening to music, or by reading something that has nothing to do with work.

If you are at school, you usually sit and use your brain during class. So, you can only balance your mind and body by using your body during break times. If you use your brain both during class and break times, it will cause an unbalanced state.

Although there are individual differences, a general rule is to have a different stimulus during break times. If you work in a very quiet place, you may want to go to a coffee shop where a little loud music is played during your lunch break. If your work is very physical, you will need to relax so that the body can rest. If you are engaged in heavy brain work, it is not desirable to play *Go*[19] or *Shōgi*[20] during your lunch break.

Yogic exercises you can do in the office

Some companies offer a daily fixed time for employees to exercise together. Here I will introduce some effective exercises you can easily perform in your own time. Please refer to Fig.27.

A stress relieving method

What is the best way to relieve stress?

When a stimulus is felt to be overstimulating, or when it is received as a forced stimulus, that becomes stress. For this reason, stress is different for everyone. There is nothing in common. Somebody who has been brought up overprotected usually worries about small matters. They cannot adapt themselves to different situations. The weaker, more immature and less experienced they are, the more stressed they will be.

So, if you want to get rid of stress, you need to have as much experience as possible. For example, if you have experienced fasting for one week, you wouldn't mind not eating for a day or two. However, if you always eat big meals and have never skipped a meal, you may feel great stress even by skipping one meal. That is why it is important to experience all sorts of difficulties. When

---

[19] A traditional board game, which is thought to have originated in China and be the world's oldest board game continuously played to the present day. The game is very popular in East Asia. *Go* is its Japanese name.

[20] A Japanese traditional board game, also known as Japanese chess.

Fig.27 Exercises you can do in the office

1 Raise your legs. While exhaling, nod your head up and down, turn side to side, and then rotate

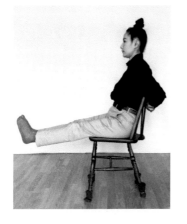

2 Cross your left leg over the right leg and twist your upper body to the left. Do the same for the other side

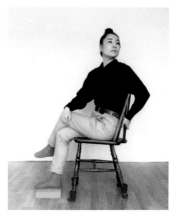

3 Raise your legs all at once. This exercise will enhance your *tanden* power and stamina

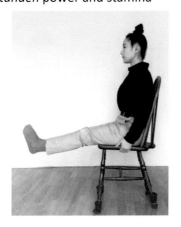

4 Circle the ankle 10 times in each direction. Do the same for the other ankle

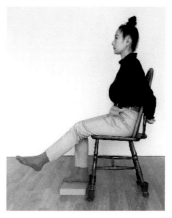

5 Raise one leg horizontally and stretch the Achilles tendon. Do the same for the other leg

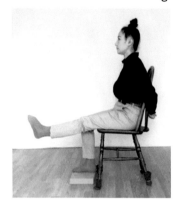

6 Shake your feet up and down

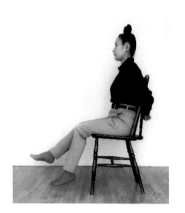

7 Hold the edge of the desk with your hands. Lean forwards keeping your heels down. Try to arch back. This will uplift and improve your feelings and enhance your concentration

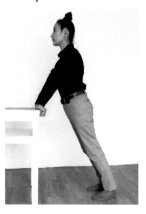

8 Hold the sides of the chair. Keeping both arms straight, raise your hips with your weight supported by the heels. Stretch the Achilles tendons. Open your chest. Look up

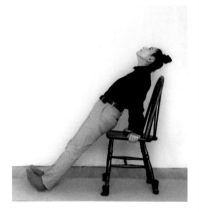

it is hot, consciously experience the hot feeling. If you turn on an air conditioner as soon as you feel hot, you may feel stressed by just a little heat and suffer from air-conditioning sickness. In other words, enhancing your adaptability is a stress relieving method.

We do not receive the harm of stress from what we enjoy. So, we should transform ourselves into somebody who can enjoy anything. We should experience what we cannot easily adapt ourselves to, or what we are not used to, so that we do not feel burdened by that stimulation next time. If we live passively or try to escape from difficulties, stress will chase us. Therefore, it is important to live a life less protected by others and less reliant on others. If we do not want to suffer, it is better to bring a little difficulty into our lives. The easier a life we pursue, the more stress will come to us.

For example, someone who has had many life-and-death experiences would be able to bear a hard situation. People who started a business with a lot of effort from nothing would not be stressed with some economic fluctuation, because they have already had bigger difficulties than that.

However, if the business owner's child or grandchild who has no experience takes over the business, they will feel tremendously burdened even with a slight change in society. They don't know how to adapt. So, the business would collapse.

There is a saying that the third generation ruins a business. This is not necessarily because of the third generation, but because of the following: the first generation becomes strong by experiencing all difficulties and so knows how to solve problems. The second and third generations, on the other hand, have an easier life due to the efforts of the first generation. They do not build the business from scratch with effort, and are instead handed the business before they are able to manage it well. They therefore tend to get stressed over even the smallest of problems.

Yoga that turns stress into enjoyment

It does not matter whether you live in a good environment or a bad environment. What matters is how you respond to things. Weak people get weaker even in good environments, and strong people get stronger even in bad environments. Depending on whether you are a weak person or a strong person, the influence of the environment will be different for each person.

The same is true of stress. Not many things cause me stress. This is because I try to turn everything into joy. I change everything to something that I can be thankful for. Some of the so-called religions teach that there is hell and paradise, happiness and unhappiness, and loss and gain. This is based on a worldly mind.

"I love my enemies, I love my allies, I make friends with pleasant people, I make friends with unpleasant people, I am grateful when I gain, I am grateful when I lose, I am happy when I pass an exam, and I am happy when I fail an exam"— this feeling of rejoicing in any situation is important.

You may ask how you can be happy when failing an exam, but it is possible to interpret this as a chance to study for another year due to the failure. If you think about it, you will understand the difference between studying for an extra year and not studying. Don't you become cleverer by studying for an extra year? If you pass immediately, you will not do any extra studying.

In that way, you should cultivate a *mind-heart that can interpret any situation in a better way, and you should train your body at the same time. This is the training of yoga. It is also a way to relieve stress. People who fuss about being stressed are demonstrating that they are weak.

Stress disappears if you can understand that someone who bullies you makes you strong. If you think you are troubled by being bullied, you will be stressed. You become a stressed person if you try to be in as little trouble as possible, try to be scolded as little as possible, and try to avoid unpleasant feelings as much as possible.

I meet unpleasant people every day. When a *dōjō* staff member comes to me and says, "Master, there is a visitor for you", I often end up listening to an unpleasant story like "My eyes are bad", "My head feels strange", or "My husband is bad. I am thinking of divorcing him".

I wonder why I have to listen to these stories from morning till evening. It is the kind of thing that would make most people a little neurotic in a week.

We human beings feel good when we see something enjoyable, but we feel bad when we see only unpleasant things. Why, then, do I not become neurotic?

The reason is simple. It is because I change these unpleasant things to objects of gratitude. Someone who says strange things is a teacher to me. "I see, I can learn that this kind of lifestyle makes this type of strange person." When we look at each thing as a teaching, we can thank everything. That is why we can feel grateful and relaxed.

"I see, lack of study can make us so stupid." We can feel grateful by thinking that this person is showing us so. "Indeed, somebody with that personality can only think in that gloomy way." We have an opportunity to learn from this.

In this way, I consider each person to be a teacher. I am grateful to each and every person. Because I receive delight from everyone and everything, I don't become neurotic or stressed.

Inability to be grateful for things comes from an underdeveloped personality and underdeveloped thinking capacity. It is from a lack of learning and studying. Please learn and study. You will be able to be grateful for so many things. The more your personality improves, the more delight and gratitude you will have for the things in your life.

Yoga is about empowering yourself from every angle.

How to change your mood through the breath

The state of our breathing, whether fast, slow, shallow, deep, strong, weak, and so on, fundamentally relates to our behaviour and psychology. By changing our breathing, we can control our behaviour and psychology. And by reading another person's breathing, we can know their inner state. We often hear the expression 'Breathe in unison with others'. This makes sense.

(1) <u>Breathing to relax well</u>
If you want to relax, breathe deeply and slowly (abdominal breathing). On the contrary, if you want to wake up, breathe fast and powerfully. Deeply inhale and deeply exhale. Yawning is 'awakening breathing'.

(2) <u>When you want to improve efficiency</u>
It is advisable to change the rhythm of your breathing from time to time. This is a way of dispersing the breath. When you need to focus on something momentarily, you hold your breath.

(3) <u>When you feel restless</u>
When you are excited or feel like complaining, breathe slowly. A big deep breath will gradually calm you down. Shallow breathing means that you are anxious or irritated. When someone is breathing in this way, it is important to wait for them to calm down. You need to have sympathy for someone with shallow breathing. If you scold them at such a time, you will make the situation worse.

(4) <u>A fighting spirit arises from powerful breathing</u>
You may sometimes feel unmotivated when trying to start work or study. At such times, it is advisable to breathe consciously and powerfully. This is because the rhythm of your breathing determines the strength of your will and movement. When you breathe powerfully, your willpower is boosted, and your movements become brisk.

Exercises to promote powerful breathing

Long, strong and deep breathing creates a life of positivity and motivation. So, using the breathing exercises shown in Fig.28, improve the opening and closing functions of your ribcage, stretch your pectoral muscles, and take in plenty of fresh oxygen.

Breathing control makes business successful

The key to dealing with a customer is to work with their breathing.
In order to attract their attention, first of all, it is necessary to have a shop front design or advertisement which makes the customer hold their breath and ask, "What is this?". I am saying this, based on the fact that we hold our breath when focused.
Next, you need something that makes them breathe out strongly for example, something that makes them feel "Wow, does something this useful exist?" or "Oh, that looks delicious!".
Furthermore, it is important not to disturb their breathing. For that purpose, you need to create an atmosphere that makes it easy to enter the shop. For example, if there are many people in the shop, it will be more welcoming.

Fig.28

Breathing exercise (1)

1 With your feet a bit wider than hip-width apart, extend your arms sideways, and open your ribcage well. Inhale slowly and deeply

2 Exhale while bringing your right hand to your right armpit and moving your left arm towards your left leg. Stretch the right side of the torso. Twist your neck to look at your left foot

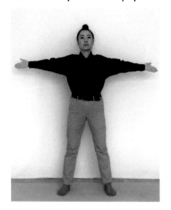

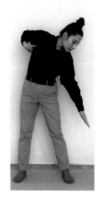

3 While inhaling, return to Step 1

4 Do the same for the other side

Breathing exercise (2)

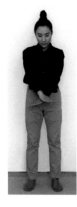

1 Open your feet hip-width apart. Exhale while crossing your arms in front and rotate them internally

2 As you inhale, put your left foot forwards and extend your arms sideways while rotating them externally

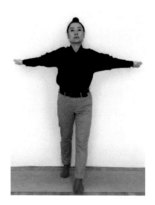

3 Do the same with the other foot

Breathing exercise (3)

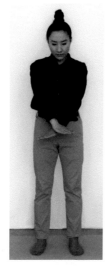

1 Open your feet hip-width apart. Exhale while crossing your arms in front and rotate them internally

2 As you inhale, put your left foot forwards and open your chest while pulling your elbows backwards and making a fist with both hands. Lift your chin up

3 Do the same with the other foot

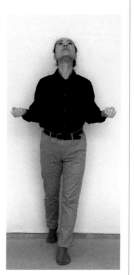

Breathing exercise (4)

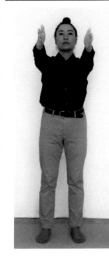

1 Open your feet hip-width apart. Inhale while extending your arms forwards

2 Exhaling while twisting your upper body left

3 Do the same for the other side

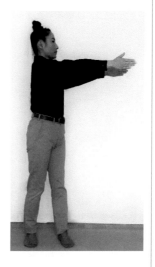

Breathing exercise (5)

1 Open your feet hip-width apart. As you exhale, move your arms backwards while rotating them internally, and bend your upper body towards your knees

2 While inhaling, straighten up your upper body, put your right foot forwards and stretch your chest with your arms extended

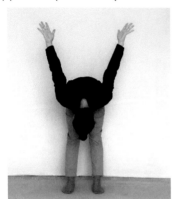

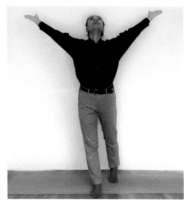

3 Do the same with the other foot

Breathing exercise (6)

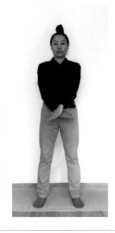

1 Open your feet hip-width apart. Exhale while crossing your arms in front and rotate them internally

2 Inhale while extending your arms diagonally upwards and rotating them externally. Lift your chin up

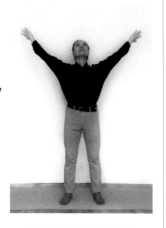

Customers like an atmosphere where they can breathe freely. So, it is important that they can breathe in their natural way. There are two types of customers: customers who are waiting to be talked to and customers who want to browse products undisturbed. For the latter type, you must pretend to be indifferent when they are looking at what they want. This is because, if they become aware of someone paying attention to them, they will be unconsciously nervous and their breathing will be disturbed. This customer is enjoying imagining the usefulness of the product by themselves. So, if it is all right to touch the product, you had better leave them alone to touch it.

When their desire for the product increases, they start holding their breath or putting strength into their breathing. At that time, you can explain the benefits of the product so that it can help them breathe more strongly. This is a service to the customer, and it is also a key to selling.

After the purchase, the customer's breathing slows down with peace of mind and joy. At that time, you must further work with this breathing. For example, you can say, "We will replace it at any time if there is a problem", or "Please use it with confidence". Then, the customer will leave the shop with that slow and relaxed breathing.

How to read books efficiently

To improve the effectiveness of your reading, first skim through the book and become aware of its content. At this time, it doesn't matter whether you understand what is written or not. Its purpose is to prepare your mind and get a sense of comfort. You will feel less resistant to what is familiar to you, and you can devote yourself to what you are comfortably interested in.

Sit in a good posture, open your eyes wide, stare at each word, read a little fast while making a long and powerful out-breath. Then you will grasp the content well.

If you read while nodding your head in agreement with each word, as if communicating with yourself, the impression of the content will become deeper so that it can stay with you longer.

If you interpret the content in your own words, it will help your interest deepen so that your concentration can increase further. The impression will become clearer, and it will be recorded in your brain as a strong memory.

If time permits, it is best to read aloud while writing something. It is because the movement of the hand directly relates to the cerebrum. When you read aloud, you can concentrate well and remember the content well.

It is a good idea to read aloud when you are distracted. Read to yourself as though you are the listener. In other words, read as if you are listening to the content and responding with agreement or disagreement. This way of reading involves your response at each point of the document, which will help you remember the content well.

How to use your eyes when reading

Read while moving your neck and shoulders from time to time. If you tense your shoulders and neck, it will cause blood congestion in those areas, which will result in poor blood circulation to your eyes.

It is also effective to read with laughter. When you laugh, your abdomen strengthens, and your breathing becomes deep. Then your body loosens, your mind relaxes, and so your eyes get less tired.

In order to read without eye strain, try different ways of reading the text. For example, it is advisable to read alternately what is written in bold and what is written in fine print.

Sometimes read while taking notes, and at other times, read aloud. Coordinating the whole body reduces the strain on the eyes.

You should change your posture when reading. For example, read while looking from the side, read alternately with one eye, and read while changing the distance between the document and your eyes. Generally, 30 cm is said to be a good distance, but there is no need to worry about this. It is much better for the eyes if you move the document closer to or farther away from them.

Change your reading speed. Read both quickly and slowly.

Focus your eyes but don't just look with your eyes. Look with your heart as if you were moved.

How to avoid occupational illness

Some professions demand us to use a particular part of the body to an extreme degree: using only your hands, lower back, eyes, and so on. If we do that, stress will accumulate there. Also, we may have to work in an extreme environment, such as in a very hot or cold place constantly. A profession which allows us to use the body and mind evenly or to work in a comfortable environment — this is a very difficult thing to hope for. Therefore, we must find a way to tolerate some undesirable working conditions.

First of all, those who regularly use one part of their body should consciously use the other parts. For example, if your work involves writing with your right hand, you should do other things with your left hand as much as possible. If you always look through a microscope at work, you should avoid tiring your eyes during holidays and at breaks and try to use your ears and whole body. In principle, these simple methods are effective.

Of course, because people who get so-called occupational illnesses have overexerted themselves, it is a prerequisite to improve their working conditions.

Work environment issues are also difficult even if we take the example of air conditioning. Whether our civilisation is too advanced or underdeveloped, it is anyhow unnatural.

When you leave an air-conditioned room, ideally you should move to a warmer place in small stages. If you walk straight into a hot place, you will surely get sick. You need to prepare and allow your body to adapt. When you stay in a cool place for a long time, your body adapts to the cold temperature. So, if you suddenly go out into the heat, your nerves and hormones will be disturbed.

When you are to return from an unbalanced state to the normal state, you should make the change slowly, which is natural. If you change suddenly, you may even die. It is very dangerous to have a person who is fasting eat a lot at once. They should return to a normal diet gradually.

However, such facilities are not always available in reality. So, when you work in an air-conditioned room, you should sometimes go out to feel the heat. Similar to alternating between hot and cold baths or having a cold shower after a hot bath, exposure to contrasting stimuli within a short time will be rather beneficial for your health.

V

Yoga in Your Home

- Make your home a yoga *dōjō*

Home is a place to relax

It may seem obvious, but a home is a place to relax. "I feel relieved when I get home"—this is natural. It is nice to have such a home.

Recently, taxi fares have risen considerably. Even when it is more economical, both in terms of time and cost, to stay at an inn or hotel than to go home by taxi at midnight, it seems that many people still go home. Even if it means spending a costly taxi fare, they probably feel more relaxed in their own home.

Yoga's view of home and work can be shown in the following flow diagram:
• Work → Tension → Devoting all your energy → For society
• Home → Relaxation → Rebuilding your strength → For yourself and family

Therefore, if your home is a place of tension, it will be a problem. Even for children, school is a place of tension. The same goes for cram schools and various kinds of after-school activities. When they are at home, children need time to relax and build up their strength for the following day. Housewives also need to be relaxed except when they are in charge of household affairs. However, they may find it more difficult to distinguish and alternate between tension and relaxation than people who have a profession.

Unless every member of the family feels comfortable at home, it would not be worth having such a place.

In society, if you make a mistake, you may be held liable. Pursuing who is responsible at home can lead to family breakdown. At home, there should be no judge or prosecutor. At home, everyone has to be each other's defender.

In society and work, you may sometimes need to be untruthful to yourself. You may have to meet people you don't like with a smile. You will also need various tactics to get a contract signed.

However, such tricks are unnecessary at home. It is at home that you can expose yourself as you are, without a mask.

If the family members are performing a masked play, it is no longer called home. The home is a place where you can forgive each other, where you can relax, and where you may fart involuntarily.

Please make use of the principles of yoga, which teach the balance of tension outside (workplace) and relaxation inside (home).

Don't scold but encourage your children

Parents raise their children. At home, they provide practical education on how to view, think about and do things. Children are mirrors of their parents. Every move and every word of the parents are transmitted to their children. For children, that is an opportunity for home-based self-study via experience.

On the other hand, children have school education, which is provided by professionals of education. Please note that the home is not a place to replay school education. You should not recreate school life at home. The home is a place of relaxation for children as well.

The role of parents is to create an environment in which children feel easy to study, and an atmosphere and stimulus that motivates children to learn. It is also their role to encourage and comfort their children. When a child has got a low mark, it should be the teacher who scolds him, not the parents. Even if the parents do not scold him, the child is aware that he has received the low mark. What the parents should do is to encourage him.

Even when people in society say, "Isn't this child a little stupid?", the parents shouldn't say the same. Instead, they should console and encourage him, saying things like 'You can do it if you try' or 'You have the ability to be a wonderful child'. The home should not be a court. There should be no prosecutor in the home. The home is a place where you comfort each other and develop your strengths.

In recent years, school education has become more and more standardised, and the method of evaluating children's abilities has also become standardised. If the parents accept it as it is, children won't be comfortable at all. It is strange if a child's evaluation is based on school grades. You must guide your children in a direction where individuals can live as they are, in their own way. It is the parents' duty to help their children lead a life that suits them.

By the way, when giving advice to your children, they will not listen if they are not convinced by your motives. Even if what you say sounds good, they will resist if you are doing it for your own sake, not for them. However, it seems that many parents give advice to their children out of their own concerns, because they are worried, they dislike something, or they are frustrated. You must eliminate these selfish thoughts in order to give compassionate education.

True love for someone is to give what is needed by and suitable for that person. The same can be said for your own self. Love for yourself is to give yourself what suits you best.

For example, let's take the case of providing love and care to flowers. If you do not use the necessary fertilisers or know the correct care for the flowers, they will die, which essentially means you do not love them. There are many instances of false love. Take cuddling a baby as an example. To cuddle a baby when you should not do so is not love but self-satisfaction. Love is to reach out with your hands when you should do so. It is not love to reach out when you shouldn't. A baby is not a toy. To cuddle them when you think they are cute and not cuddle them at all when you don't want to do so — this is selfish.

Anyway, please make sure that your home is a place to relieve the tension you experience in the outside world. Now, let's look at what yoga teaches about eating, exercising, bathing and sleeping.

Ask your body what to eat

'To live' can be understood as repeatedly taking in energy and expending it by moving and thinking, using oneself as a medium. How one moves and thinks is the content of that person's life.

Of all the ways to take in energy, people are most interested in food, or nutrition. Since yoga emphasises oxygen intake as much as nutrition, breathing techniques have been researched as mentioned in earlier chapters. But here, I will pay deeper attention to the diet which I mentioned in Chapter 2.

Many books are published on nutrition or food. It is hard to decide what method to follow. Broadly speaking, they can be categorised into ① those based on personal experience, ② those based on academic studies, and ③ those combining the two. Each type has its advantages and disadvantages.

In my view, I have doubts about putting full confidence in personal experience ① when it comes to nutrition.

When I went to a boarding junior high school, the quality of the meals was very poor, compared to the richness of my meals at home, so that I, even as a child, wondered if it was all right. Even so, my health was better there than it had been at home. Of course, health is not completely determined by diet.

Next, when I went to the mainland of China during prewar military training, I was forced to eat a lot. Because I had to journey further inland and needed to be able to go without food for some time, I was forced to practise eating big meals. And I became able to eat nearly one *shō*[21] of rice at one time.

In other words, according to environment and training, we can adapt ourselves to a diet whether poor in quality or large in quantity. This is also called 'habit'.

After the war, I went to India to practise yoga. Most of the Indians who practised yoga were pure vegetarians and I followed their way, but the neighbouring Pakistanis had a diet based on meat. In terms of health, there were no differences between Indians and Pakistanis. After that, I also experienced a life with only Chinese food and a life with only Western food. Also, at some time, I was a member of various dietary *dōjō*s.

The reason I tried so many dietary ways was because my physical condition was extremely unstable, and I hoped some diet would help my physical condition. People with weak gastrointestinal tracts are more concerned about food and drink than others. I had the same motive. I also tried primitive natural foods and strange, bizarre foods. However, there was no dietary method that suited me perfectly.

The second category ② is based on academic studies. The weakest point here is that theories are uncertain, and we do not know when they will change. What was said to be right yesterday may be corrected tomorrow by today's new discovery. It used to be said that cholesterol was bad, but nowadays it is said that there is good cholesterol and bad cholesterol. It is worrying to follow a theory blindly when it may change at any time.

Also, I am not happy with academic nutritional theories because they lack actual experience. These theories see food just as physical matter that is separate from the human body. Food and nutrition are not the same. Food can be 'alive or dead', depending

---

[21] A Japanese traditional unit to measure volume. One *shō* equals about 1.8 litres.

on different combinations. I also disagree that academic nutritional theories still give central importance to calories.

The third category ③ is the combination of experience and academics. However, it is not so easy to support empirical facts with academic explanation. Also, one person's experience is not always valid for others.

For example, it is said in Japan, "Don't mix alcoholic drinks". However, in a Western meal, they take different drinks before, during and after a meal. Mixing alcohol is a daily occurrence for them. Even among Japanese people, some start with beer, then have *sake*[22] and drink whiskey later. Others stick with *shōchū*[23] from beginning to end. If the amount of alcohol is the same, which way is wrong? Probably no one can clearly answer in academic terms.

This is not a serious problem. So, let's put it aside and go to the conclusion. That is, "Your body knows what food suits you. Listen to your body. Follow your body."

In yoga, it is said to 'live by individuality'. This also applies to diet. So, we should eat according to our individuality. Nowadays, we eat according to advertisements and information too often. Besides, we are not our natural 'self'. This is where the problem arises. Many people don't know what their true needs are.

Increase nutrition by combining ingredients

What is a truly correct diet? Yoga teaches this with the phrase 'Ask your inner wisdom'.

---

[22] A Japanese brewed alcoholic beverage made from fermented rice.
[23] A Japanese distilled alcoholic beverage made from sweet potato, barley, rice or other ingredients. *Shōchū* has a higher alcohol percentage than *sake*.

Animals eat according to their true needs based on their inner wisdom. They adopt a diet that enhances their innate ability, that is, a natural diet.

However, the human diet is based on processed foods. We do not only eat for survival like animals, but also for enjoyment. So, it is easy for the human diet to become unnatural.

When we repeatedly do the same thing in any area of our life, not only in our diet, we become addicted. The power of this habit (unnatural power) suppresses our inner wisdom (natural power), and we come to not know what our true needs are. People who take three meals a day feel like eating three times, and people who eat snacks want snacks. However, in reality, this desire in us is habitual and often does not match our true needs.

In yoga, we do the following as a method to discover our true needs and a diet that suits us:
① Break eating habits by fasting.
② Increase natural responses by eating basic foods (raw food, whole food). This is called a natural diet.

Basic food is referred to as 'staple food', which develops your natural desire and lets you know what kind of processed foods are suitable for you as complementary foods.

Because we humans have a social life, we cannot always eat when we want. Therefore, it often happens that, even when we don't need to eat, we eat because it's time to eat or because we are socialising. 'Overeating' does not simply refer to quantity but indicates that we eat when we don't need to. When we have to eat in this way, we should consciously create the desire to eat, and then eat.

Next, let's talk about the dietary wisdom that yoga teaches us.

As I have said many times, the basic idea is a small meal of diverse foods.

(1) Balanced cooking methods

Unlike animals, we humans cook. We need a sense of balance in how to cook: how to apply heat, how to combine different foods, and so on. The more methods we use the better. The best way to apply heat is by 'steaming', followed by 'stir-frying in oil'. Good food combinations are 'roots and leaves', 'both the skins and the flesh of fruits' and 'meat and bone'.

For example, if you don't eat whole soybeans, a key is to eat tofu and soy pulp at the same time. Meat stew with bones is better than steak.

(2) The effect of food combination

When you cook rice with soybeans, the protein is equivalent to milk. When soybeans are added to wheat, the amount of essential amino acids increases, and when wheat is added to rice, the balance of yin and yang increases. The synergistic effect enhances the nutritional power.

Also, adding vegetable protein to animal protein, adding vegetable fat to animal fat, or adding seaweeds to vegetables will reduce any harmful effects from either and enhance the nutritional power of both.

However, I don't mean that any combination will do. For example, it is known that adding white sugar to something destroys its important minerals, vitamins and amino acids.

Now I will give you an example of good combinations with rice:
▪ Rice with adzuki beans. The protein of adzuki beans is three times that of rice. Adzuki's starch is of good quality, and it is rich in vitamins and minerals.
▪ Rice with foxtail millet. Foxtail millet is rich in fat and vitamin B.
▪ Rice with Japanese barnyard millet. Japanese barnyard millet has lysine, which is an essential amino acid.

▪ Rice with radish leaves. Radish leaves have three times as much vitamin A as eel, twice as much vitamin B as cow's milk, and twice as much vitamin C and minerals as mandarin oranges.

If rice is your staple food, please refer to these points and maintain balance in your diet.

'Energy sustaining foods' are good foods for the intestines and liver

Stamina is usually understood as a capacity for endurance. One can say it is physical fitness that keeps you from running out of breath too quickly, that is, lasting physical strength. As we all know, this is best in adolescence. The middle-aged compensate for physical strength with experience and mental strength. It is said that adolescents have stamina because their intestines and liver work very actively. From this, we can say that foods that are good for the intestines and liver, in other words, foods that are high in vitamins and minerals, are stamina foods.

You can roughly guess whether a food is good for stamina by eating a small amount and seeing if it fills you up and keeps you going for a long time. Examples of such foods are brown rice rather than white rice, raw vegetables rather than boiled vegetables, wild grasses rather than vegetables, stir-fried foods rather than boiled foods, and roots rather than leaves.

Stamina foods include Chinese pearl barley, aloe, sesame seeds, black beans, snails, seaweeds, bitter summer oranges, salt, smoked fish, chameleon plant, yam, garlic, walnuts, spring onions, eels, tree buds, and vegetable oil. All of these purify the blood, warm the body, soothe the mind, and become the source of stamina. A person with a warm mind and body has stamina. A person with strong intestines and liver has a warm body.

Besides nutrition, the intake of oxygen is also important. Long-distance runners have excellent cardiorespiratory function, which means they have a strong ability to take in oxygen.

The most necessary thing for the brain is oxygen. If your breath becomes short by vigorous exercise, it is because your whole body demands much more oxygen. Physical training and deep breathing can improve your oxygen intake and use. You will be able to take in a lot and use a little.

Raw vegetables are good stamina foods because they contain a lot of oxygen. Eating raw vegetables means eating oxygen.

In this way, you can increase stamina by combining good nutrition and exercise. You also need to consider stamina from the following perspective:

For athletes, for example, the balance between stamina and power is important, although its degree depends on the sport which each athlete is engaged in. Even a long-distance runner cannot win just by having high cardiorespiratory endurance. Power is also required for the last spurt to outperform other runners. Having stamina in the true sense means having both endurance and instantaneous power.

You need foods that increase the flexibility of the muscles, strengthen the bones, and raise the body temperature. These foods include yang vegetables (seaweeds, root vegetables and so on) and meat.

Eating meat warms your body immediately and gives you more power but acidifies the blood when you exercise. So, to balance this, you should put alkaline foods in your main diet and then add meat as needed. Professional athletes should be physically flexible as a result of training, but in reality, many of them are stiff because of eating too many animal products. I have to say that this is due to an unbalanced diet.

Use your brain more to improve its function

If certain foods improved brain function, most people would eat them. However, aside from science fiction, there cannot really be such things.

Although we cannot say that something improves our brain function for certain, there is a way to stop it declining.

There is research showing that many children with so-called low IQ were born from mothers who were deficient in calcium, B vitamins, protein and so on. In other words, foods containing these may be indispensable for the nutrition of the brain.

It used to be said that glutamic acid should be taken to improve brain function, as it was a highly abundant nutrient in the brain. However, there are strong barriers that limit the entry of substances into the brain to ensure that only the required amounts enter. Even if you take a lot of glutamic acid, not all of it can cross the barriers to enter the brain.

Returning to the subject of nutrition, there are some foods that contain a lot of essential nutrients for the brain as noted above. These are beans, spring onions, green vegetables, fruits, egg yolk, liver, butter, cheese, tomatoes and so on.

However, it is more important to use the brain than worrying about nutrition. Every part of the human body will deteriorate if it is not used. The same is true for the brain.

Other factors that interfere with brain function include poor blood circulation, lack of oxygen, constant excitement and poor posture. So, it is important to eliminate these adverse conditions first. In this sense, light exercise and good posture are essential for brain function.

Additionally, foods containing vitamin A and calcium are good for frustration, vitamin B and sodium are good for laziness, vitamin K for timidness, and vitamin C and calcium for restlessness. These foods will help such conditions improve.

The appetite centre, located in the cerebrum, is close to the centre for sexual drive and the centre for emotions. So, they are interrelated. People who can control their appetite also have easier control over their sexual drive and emotions. When the appetite is disturbed, the emotions and sexual drive are also disturbed.

How to find your ideal weight

Broadly speaking, there are two misunderstandings about obesity. One of them is due to standard weight. The other is due to the impression given by appearance. Whether one's appearance is deemed fat or slim is a matter of subjectivity, and so I will not discuss that here.

Essentially, each person has one good value for their weight. There is no standard weight. There is the average weight of a group of people, which you can get by adding everybody's weight and dividing it by the number of people in the group.

Let's forget about saying that you are obese because you are heavier than the standard weight, or that you are thin because you are lighter than the standard weight. The optimal weight for you is the weight that enables you to be at your best. At that weight, you feel good, move lightly, and have stamina.

One *sumō* wrestler said, "When I was active, I weighed more than 130 kilograms. But now, ten years after I retired, I'm in the 90-kilogram range. I was not flabby at 130 kilograms. My body had necessary muscles and fat, which were like a hard iron plate." If he weighed 130 kilograms even after retirement, he might be considered obese. Obesity is generally a condition in which unwanted fat (or water and so on) remains in the body and causes illness. *Sumō* wrestlers' fat is not unhealthy.

The difference between these two types of fat is that unhealthy fat is soft, burns easily and is susceptible to bacterial infection while healthy fat is hard, does not burn easily and is gained through exercise and training. Accumulating fat through exercise and training requires lots of effort. The most problematic cause of obesity is this build-up of unhealthy fat (fat due to overnutrition). It can also be caused by poor excretion.

The body tries to eliminate unnecessary things, but if it cannot excrete fully for some reason, the remaining substances will be

---

Fig.29 Abnormalities in the body that can be detected by the way unhealthy fat builds up

Flabby arms indicate abnormalities of the shoulders, neck or head.

A fleshy lower back indicates postural overstraining in this area, or abnormalities of the liver or stomach.

Excess fat in the abdomen indicates intestinal abnormalities, looseness and congestion of the internal organs, or prolapse.

A large upper leg indicates abnormalities of Lumbar 1 or 2, bladder, stomach, intestines, liver or caecum.

A large lower leg indicates abnormalities of Lumbar 4 or 5, defecation, large intestine, prostate, or lower limbs.

stored in the body to prevent them affecting the cells of other organs. An example of this is swelling by water retention.

To get rid of this unhealthy fat, you need to reduce food intake or increase your physical activity. This is the main measure. People who are fat and tend to have constipation have poor excretion, and so they need to eat something that improves excretion.

The next issue is where the unhealthy fat accumulates in the body. By seeing where your residual energy is stored, you can know what part of your body is not functioning well. This is a worse state than putting on fat just by overeating.

Exercises you can easily do while watching television

If you live an inactive lifestyle, your muscles will become stiff. But that doesn't mean you must consider doing any special exercise. Rather, you had better devise ways to move your body diligently in your daily life. For example, even while watching television, you have opportunities to train your muscles. If you can do this daily, many times a day, you will be able to avoid the stigma of being a 'lethargic person'.

Bodybuilding without equipment can be done anytime, anywhere. For example, without using an expander, you can perform the same pulling action and still exert the same force on your body as if you were using one. Also, it is similarly effective to perform the weightlifting action with full strength as if you were doing it with a weight. *Sumō* wrestlers' *shiko*[24] gives you the same effect. You may overdo muscle training using equipment such as barbells and dumbbells, because the results can be seen even in

---

[24] One of the basic *sumō* exercises in which a wrestler raises a leg high in the air to the side and then brings it down with a stomp.

Fig.30

Exercise you can do while watching television (1)

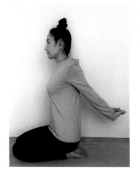

Interlace your fingers behind you. With your arms raised to maximum height, hold your breath. Swing your arms up and down 10 times and left to right 10 times

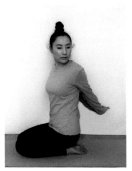

Exercise you can do while watching television (2)

1 Stretch up your arms with fingers interlaced and palms turned out. While exhaling, bend your upper body forwards

2 While exhaling, bend your upper body sideways

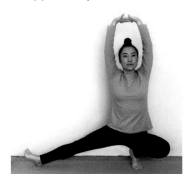

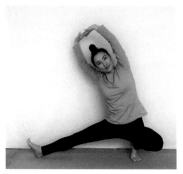

3 (right) While exhaling, bend your upper body towards the straightened leg

Do the same for the other side.

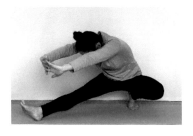

an unexpectedly short time. So, please keep in mind, as the main principle, that you must organise this training to improve the functionality of the entire body in good balance. While training, you can consciously change angles, exert more or less power, stretch and contract, and so on.

Exercise you can do while watching television (3)

1 Pull your elbows backwards. Stretch your chest

2 While inhaling, close your elbows and lift your hips

3 While exhaling, turn your hips right and twist your upper body left. Open your elbows

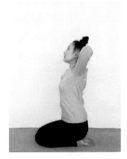 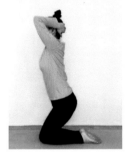 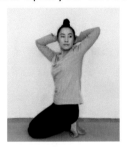

Exercise you can do while watching television (4)

1 Place your thumbs on the arches of your feet. Exhale

2 While inhaling, lift your chin up towards the ceiling

3 While exhaling, lift up your hips and raise your chest and belly

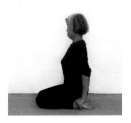 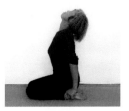 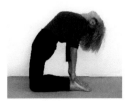

Exercise you can do while watching television (5)

1 Shake your legs up and down, and sideways

2 Bend your upper body 3 times

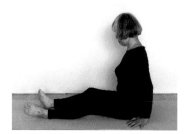

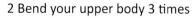

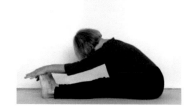

3 Bend your right leg, place your right foot outside your left knee. Bring your left elbow outside the right knee. While exhaling, twist your torso and neck to the right. Do the same for the other side

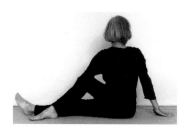

Exercises to strengthen your body in daily life

(1) For ankles and knees

It has long been said that people with strong legs are physically and mentally strong. To make your legs strong, it is important to make your knees and ankles strong. The strength of the knees is a manifestation of the strength of the lower back and abdomen. It is alarming if your knees begin to weaken. Stronger knees help your neck be stronger and brain waves be more stable.

The ability to flex and extend the knees correlates with the ability to open and close the pelvis, which correlates with breathing power. Breathing power correlates with will power. To strengthen the knees, it is essential to strengthen the ankles, both of which relate to the strength of the internal organs and the blood circulation in the brain as well as throughout the body. To strengthen your ankles and knees, please do the following exercises daily:

① Instead of using a lift, go up and down the stairs two steps at a time.

② Run up a slope.

③ In *seiza*, sit with strength in your knees and heels and stretch your back and neck, which will strengthen your legs. To put strength in your knees and heels, lower down your pelvis and tighten your hip muscles and anal muscles.

④ If you hold your knees or use some support while moving to sit down, your legs will weaken. In other words, aging is accelerated. To prevent this, practice maintaining a half-squatting position.

⑤ When walking, do not walk lazily, but walk fast. Measure the time for the route you walk every day and try to shorten the time little by little. This will help your legs become stronger. It is also good to set a goal and try to walk that distance fast in one breath.

(2) For a weak stomach

Modern people who use their nerves a lot tend to suffer from gastrointestinal disorders. In particular, Japanese people seem to have a weak gastrointestinal tract. Abdominal breathing and acupressure can be effective to strengthen the function of the autonomic nerves. From the same perspective, the following exercises will be good to do two or three times a day, avoiding the time directly after meals: Open both legs in a standing position, lean slightly forwards, draw your abdomen and stomach in as far as you can, and hold for 6 seconds with the feeling that they are attached to your back. It is a problem if they do not move with your intention.

(3) <u>Increasing your grip strength is good for the brain</u>
The hands and brain are related. If you don't want your brain to weaken, you need to increase your grip strength.

When you do press-ups, try to support your body with your fingers instead of your palms. Hanging on a horizontal bar or grabbing a ball tightly is also good. It will also be good to wring a large wet item such as a sheet with your hands or carry your shopping bag with one or two fingers. If you try to consciously put some burden on your fingers, it will be quite helpful in reducing the decline in your brain function.

Bathing as a method for improving health

Do you like a hot or lukewarm bath? Depending on the temperature of the bath, the effect will be completely different.

If you stay in lukewarm water for a long time, first your muscles will loosen. When the muscles relax, hormone secretion improves, nerve balance is restored, tension is released, and excitement subsides. Also, since it alkalises the blood, it is effective even when the blood is acidified by eating too much meat or sweet food.

If you soak in hot water for a short time, the heat generated in your body will make you feel better, and your ability to sweat and excrete will increase. Also, blood circulation will improve rapidly, as is well known.

The big difference between hot and lukewarm baths is that the former stimulates the sympathetic nerves and the latter stimulates the parasympathetic nerves. In other words, when you want to start off doing something, a hot bath will awaken you and tighten your muscles nicely. On the other hand, lukewarm water is good before going to sleep because it relaxes you. If you stay in hot water for a long time, you will get tired. A quick dip into lukewarm water has no particular effect.

Taking a cold shower or bath has a similar effect as taking a hot bath. That is to say, it tightens the muscles and nerves and enhances the function of the sympathetic nerves. A cold bath that cools a warm body is very effective in tightening the body and mind. Even with this benefit, cooling your warm body suddenly is dangerous. You should soak your toes, which are the farthest from your heart, and then soak other parts, gradually approaching the area of the heart.

Cold baths can be taken all year round, but if you are new to them, it is a good idea to start in the summer. Get used to cold baths gradually, instead of starting without good preparation in a cold season. For inexperienced people, the water may feel cold. However, it won't be hard if you focus your mind on the *tanden* and put strength into your out-breath. It is also a good idea to take a cold bath with determined gusto. It will be great if you come to feel good with this form of bathing. A cold bath after working hard can be most enjoyable.

The bathing time is usually a few seconds to a few minutes, or as long as you don't feel uncomfortably cold. To increase the effect, rub or brush your skin in the water to activate the reaction of the blood vessels.

In a cold bath, first the blood vessels of the skin constrict, then the skin becomes pale and gets goosebumps. Over time, the blood vessels dilate, the skin becomes pink and the metabolism speeds up. However, because a cold bath gives a strong stimulation and lowers the surface temperature of your body, you may need to warm your limbs afterwards. If you take a cold bath every day, your skin will quickly respond to sudden changes in temperature. Starting in the summer will especially help to train your body and prevent illness.

It is better to take a cold bath with your whole body, but you can just immerse your hands and feet in cold water. This partial cold bath may be better for the elderly and people with palpitations or hyperthyroidism.

In addition to training the skin, it is also good for people with a weak constitution and people who are prone to catching a cold. A cold bath is also effective for psychosomatic diseases such as autonomic imbalance, bronchial asthma and angina, as well as digestive diseases such as chronic constipation, muscular rheumatism, diabetes and obesity. It strengthens the function of the skin and helps to promote and maintain health.

Yogic exercises for good sleep

The life force functions with the alternating rhythm of yang and yin, work and rest, tension and relaxation. You have to consider this rhythm for physical and mental health. For example, if you only think of eating food but forget about excreting, your approach to nutrition will be incomplete.

The nerves function well when the sympathetic nervous system and the parasympathetic nervous system work well alternately. If the sympathetic nervous system functions at its best during daytime, you can apply your full capacity at work, and if the parasympathetic nervous system functions dominantly during nighttime, you can sleep peacefully.

In other words, if you keep your body and mind tense during the day by working hard, the opposite state, namely relaxation, will come to you at night so that you will sleep soundly. Therefore, you must fully burn your energy for your work during the day. If you are lazy during daytime, you may not be able to sleep well.

However, in our modern lifestyle, we may not be using our body fully. In olden days, people used both body and mind fully. Nowadays, many people are coming to use almost only brain and *mind-heart. It is no exaggeration to say that this is causing 'insomnia'. Did hunters in ancient times suffer from insomnia? Rather, I think they would keep a night watch against dangers while rubbing their drowsy eyes.

What can we do to fall asleep smoothly after unbalanced daytime activities? First of all, I suggest 'yogic exercises for good sleep'. These aim to alleviate stiffness from various areas of the body. Please try any of the exercises shown in Fig.31. Even if you are somebody who sleeps soundly, do give it a go. You will be able to sleep much more deeply, and so will awaken differently.

Another method to enter the sleep state is to induce it by suggestion, saying 'I am going to sleep'. If you still cannot sleep, do not sleep till you feel sleepy. It causes an unnatural state if you try to sleep when not feeling sleepy. Even if you wake up at midnight, why should you not stay up until you feel sleepy again?

The environment you sleep in is also important. I suggest you use a hard futon rather than a soft bed. Then, your spine will avoid becoming distorted, and so you will have a better sleep.

A warm bath dilates your blood vessels and relaxes your body and nerves, and so you will get a good sleep. However, a very hot or cold bath will stimulate you to stay awake.

Cold bedding tightens your body and causes difficulty for going to sleep. Bedding should be warm to encourage good sleep.

The state of your eyeballs also relates to your sleep very much. In order to fall asleep, stick out your eyeballs and turn them upwards. This loosens the body from the shoulders and up. Drawing the eyeballs inwards is a stimulus to cause tension.

Tossing about in your sleep means that you are moving to adjust your body after the unnatural ways of using it during the daytime.

So, please do not worry. Children, especially, toss and turn a lot during sleep. They regain balance in this way. It is proof of an excellent ability to recover naturally.

Fig.31

Exercise for good sleep (1)

1 Shake your legs. With palms facing up, move your arms upwards while shaking them

2 Rotate the arms internally and externally. While shaking, move them down

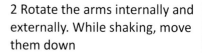

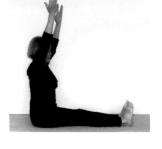

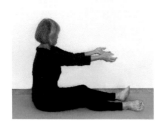

Exercise for good sleep (2)

1 (right) While exhaling, bend your upper body forwards and grab your toes

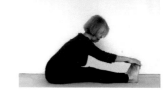

2 Put the soles of your feet together. Pull them towards your body

3 While exhaling, rock your body back and forth, and side to side

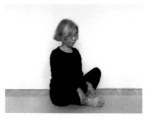

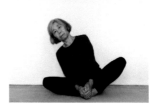

Exercise for good sleep (3)

1 Put your palms together
and exhale

2 While inhaling, extend your
arms upwards. Raise your gaze to
the ceiling and hold your breath

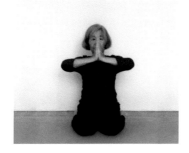

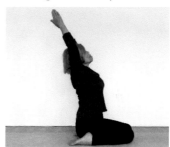

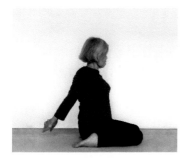

3 (left) While exhaling, lower your
arms to your sides and then
interlace your fingers behind you

4 While inhaling, bend your
upper body forwards
with your chin out

5 While exhaling fully, raise your
hips and extend your arms with
your forehead on the floor

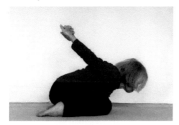

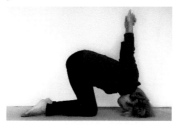

Exercise for good sleep (4)

1 Open your feet and knees hip-width apart. Keep the width. While exhaling, bend your body backwards, raise your chest, and push your abdomen and waist area forwards.

2 Turn your face from side to side

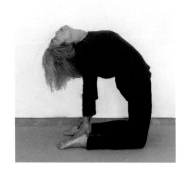

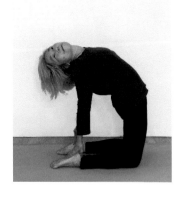

3 While inhaling, pull your chin in

4 While exhaling, lower your hips down

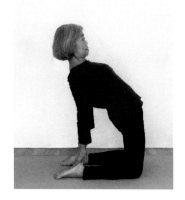

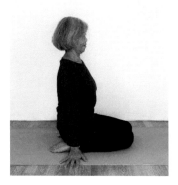

VI

Meditation Discipline Leads You to the State of *Mu*

- How to deepen and expand the self

Rāja-yoga, the principal training of yoga

Considering that we can only see and comprehend things according to our own capacity and level of experience, I might be unqualified to talk about *Meditation.

Masters or experts of *Meditation are Christ, Shakyamuni, Muhammad, Nichiren, Dōgen, and so on. Studies on how these great saints in human history disciplined their mind, body and lifestyle tell us that they commonly practised the *Meditation *discipline of yoga. I wish I could learn from them and be saved.

The first four stages of yoga teach the prerequisites of *Meditation as preparatory training. Otherwise, it would be very difficult. Training of breathing and *discipline of the *mu-mind (*mushin) are particularly necessary.

The significance of *Meditation is to grasp the truth through feeling and thinking about things broadly, deeply, highly and reverently.

For example, please imagine a situation where you meet somebody. Ordinarily, you regard the situation as happening only in that place at that time. However, from the perspective of *Meditation, you could not have met that person unless all events and occurrences had happened from your ancestral time to the present time, and unless all conditions had come to be for that encounter. Furthermore, from all the people in the whole world, the two of you have been selected to meet.

Also, when we encounter good teachings and receive benefits from useful things, we cannot help but think that it is due to the efforts of our numerous ancestors over the long history.

In this way, it is only when we have a truthful *mind-heart, which can feel all of the visible and invisible blessings, that we can comprehend things correctly. Then the essential qualities of a *religious *mind-heart naturally arise: unconditional gratitude, self-reflective repentance, humbleness with respect, devoted service, and practising love (*kansha, zange, geza, hōshi, aigyō*).

I think you have understood that *Meditation *discipline is the basic *discipline to attain a correct *mind-heart, take the right actions and attain a *religious *mind-heart. Originally, yoga *discipline refers only to this *Meditation *discipline. The preparatory training to create a suitable mind and body for that is 'hatha-yoga' (*yama, niyama, āsana, prānāyāma, pratyāhāra*), and the main training is 'rāja-yoga'.

'Rāja-yoga' is the unified training of the following phases: to unite the mind and body (*dhāranā*), to create the most stable state of the mind and body (*dhyāna*), to empty the *mind-heart from all attachments (*bhakti*), to connect oneself with others (*samādhi*), to enlighten the *busshō (*buddhi*), and to be in true joy (*prasāda*).

When we train ourselves by applying *hatha-yoga* and *rāja-yoga* in our daily life, it becomes 'daily life yoga' (*karma-yoga*).

Let's start looking into *dhāranā*.

Dhāranā (concentration) — the fifth stage

This *discipline begins with concentration of attention and concentration of consciousness. These two types of concentration require relaxation, deep and even breathing, and a mind that easily becomes single-focused. When these conditions are met, the ability to sense and think becomes stronger.

When you are lying down and relaxing, even a small sound will sound loud. Also, when you are impressed, surprised, interested, in need of something, or under pressure, you can naturally concentrate your mind. So, the key is to consciously create such conditions.

Concentration of attention can be called 'concentration training through the body'. For example, focus your vision on something. If your eyes get tired, you can close them. However, to avoid interrupting your concentration, focus your mind on the afterimages behind your eyelids.

If you want to focus your hearing on something, it is better to choose a monotonous rhythm, such as the ticking of a clock, a flowing river, or the sound of waves.

Yoga most commonly uses a mantra method by concentrating attention on the sound of *Om* (a sacred sound). You should first chant the sound aloud as long as the out-breath lasts while you concentrate on it, and then chant it in your *mind-heart while similarly paying attention to it. *Om*, as it is a simple monosyllable, has the effect of quietening the mind and is useful for mental concentration. So, I would recommend it. Repeatedly chanting *Om* will help your mind and body calm down.

Buddhist chanting has a similar effect. However, if you don't do it in the correct posture, there may be some adverse effects caused by abnormal excitement.

In any case, while you concentrate with your ears, you had better close your eyes. Once you reach a state of 'seeing but not seeing', there is no need to worry about closing your eyes or not.

Another method of focusing attention is to concentrate your power on a part of the body. The most common way is to concentrate on the lower abdomen or navel. This includes breathing practice and training of the *tanden*, and so there are multiple effects. You should fully pay attention to your out-breath and in-breath and continue breathing rhythmically. Open your chest, pull your shoulder blades closer, level your shoulders, and then relax. To relax your shoulders, it is important to relax your hands. When the hands are tense, the shoulders become tense. If a disturbing thought arises, you must wait for it to disappear.

Concentration of consciousness is concentration training through the mind. To do this, you should concentrate on an abstract idea. You may have heard of a Zen *kōan* (公案). For example, keep thinking about 'What is nothingness?', or something impossible to understand by thinking. It is a way to get out of thinking by continuing to think about a subject that cannot be grasped even if you think about it. As concentration progresses, consciousness and senses become sharper and clearer, and at the same time, the mind becomes calmer and more relaxed.

The reason for this is as follows: concentration triggers the excitatory tension force, which then induces the inhibitory relaxation force. Conversely, the relaxing force induces the tensing force. This is Nature's law, that is, the law of life.

This highest state of balance between tension and relaxation is the highest stable state. This state is called *dhyāna*, or *zenjō* (禅定), the sixth stage. This is the origin of Japanese Zen.

The key to practising concentration, as well as *zenjō*, and the key to improving efficiency in study and work, are the same. That is, to engage yourself in things with neither tension nor slackness. For example, when you do something with tension, unnecessary resistance arises against it and interferes with concentration.

The brain has many scattered spots which get excited or inhibited according to different stimuli. Therefore, if you continue to concentrate your attention and consciousness on only one thing, as the level of excitement increases due to the intensive stimulation, the many scattered inhibitory points in the other parts of the brain will cooperate to oppose the single point of excitement. This is the state of maximum excitement with maximum calmness.

On the other hand, in a distracted state, the excitatory points and inhibitory points are scattered in many different places, which is a so-called split state. If this persists, it will cause fatigue and interfere with both concentration and relaxation.

For example, if you think you must sleep, that thought itself generates excitatory stimulation, which will make it harder to sleep. On the other hand, if you either do not seek anything or concentrate on only one thing, say, repeatedly counting numbers, it will put you to sleep before you know it. This is because you feel relaxed. This is also why you can concentrate on your work most easily when you do it with an empty mind, rather than when tensely thinking about what you must do.

The *mu*-mind (*mushin*) is a mind that does not get caught up in anything else, that is, a mind with which you do things as if you do nothing. This state of mind is called non-attachment or natural mind. It is the correct state of mind.

Dyhāna (*zenjō*) — the sixth stage

There are static and dynamic ways to practise *dhyāna*. The eyes may be closed, half open or fully open. Here I will describe the practice with closed eyes.

When practising *dhyāna* with your eyes closed, try to consciously pull your eyeballs back into your head. At this time, you need to pull your chin in and stretch the back of your neck. If the chin sticks out, the eyeballs protrude. When the eyeballs protrude, your strength is lost. Consciously protruding the eyeballs will help you sleep. And if you loosen and round your lower back, you will become sleepy. As such, sleepiness during meditation or lectures is caused by a lack of strength in the lower back and protruded eyeballs.

Consciously stretch the back of your neck and create space between the skull and the neck. Your awareness will become clearer. It is because this posture stimulates the nerves that awaken the body. To always keep the chin pulled in, bear in mind the following three things: First, create the feeling of being pulled upwards by the hair. This feels as if the top of your head were sticking up towards the sky. Second, expand your chest and push it upwards, as well as push your hips downwards. Third, stretch the rectus abdominis muscle vertically, and extend the lower back as if pushing it forwards.

When you consciously apply these three things, strength can naturally come into the *tanden*. When strength is in the *tanden*, the anal muscles tighten. When the anal muscles tighten, the spine stretches and becomes strong. At the same time, the chest and upper body naturally relax.

The *tanden* is the unification point for maintaining balance. The stronger the forces converge in the *tanden*, the more stable the body becomes, which brings greater stability to the brain. In other words, physical training is directly linked to mental cultivation.

By the way, the optimum state of mind, body, and lifestyle is that in which the opposite forces and functions, such as negative energy and positive energy, yin and yang, centrifugal force and centripetal force, use and absorption, are in the highest cooperation and unification. This state of balance between yin and yang is the natural state.

Within the body, the spine has the yang role, and the muscles have the yin role. Therefore, it is necessary and natural that the spine is as strong as possible and that the muscles are as relaxed as possible. If the spine lacks strength and the muscles are tense, they will be in an unnatural state. This state creates abnormalities.

Consciously pull your eyeballs back into the head, pull your chin in, and feel as if your head were being pulled up from above. Then relax your muscles as if you were letting them lean against the spine. To consciously relax your body, you can do autosuggestion.

For example, you can suggest to yourself that your head is relaxed, your hands are relaxed and so on, also imagining that you are in that state (visualisation). Then it will happen in that way.

Bhakti (*mushin*) — the seventh stage

Dhyāna is the *discipline of stability through the body, whereas *bhakti* is the *discipline of stability through the mind to create a peaceful mind. *Bhakti* means 'to offer oneself to another'. This is the *discipline of faith to practise surrendering oneself to God (the truth) or leaving one's fate in Nature's hands.

We unconsciously and instinctively tend to be egocentric and self-centered. This egocentrism is the cause of sins. As long as we are preoccupied with our own self, we cannot be in harmony with others or live in *samādhi*, the eighth stage, which is the state of oneness between oneself and others. In *bhakti*, we practise unconditional service to others as a *discipline to extinguish the selfish mind. The conditional mind is called 'evil desire', and this mind gives rise to complaints, anger, cursing, hatred and so on. This mind wants things to be done in self-serving ways, which is against nature. Here, peace of mind cannot be maintained.

The unconditional and attachment-free mind is called 'the mind of *hōge* (放下)' or *mushin*. In this stable and peaceful state, our mind works at its best.

Samādhi (*sanmai*) — the eighth stage

Samādhi means that one becomes united with another. That is, one's mind and the other's mind become one. For example, you can become united with your work. There is no conflict or misunderstanding here. It is a world where you and others exist together in harmony.

When you cultivate the ability to grasp things correctly through *dhyāna*, as well as the ability to accept things just as they are through *bhakti*, and when you can then unite your *mind-heart with the other's *mind-heart, the state of *samādhi* will arise. Only when you correctly grasp the other's *mind-heart can you practise 'love'. So, *samādhi* is the key to living and acting correctly. Only when you are united with your work can you truly work. Also, you will receive joy from the work. Then, working becomes a method of promoting health and a path to enlightenment.

Buddhi (enlightenment of the *busshō*) — the ninth stage

The *busshō* is a quality given only to human beings, which is the ability to drive evolution and revere all things as sacred. Unless this quality fully functions, we cannot attain the joy of living or the joy of working.

Shakyamuni and Christ found God and light in everything. They interpreted and treated everything as sacred. Only with our *mind-heart sanctified[25] can our personality be developed. Only with a sanctified *mind-heart can we have a mind of reverence, true gratitude and joy.

---

[25] The word 'sanctified' is the most direct and literal translation of the original Japanese text. However, this word might invoke in some readers an impression derived from their personal or cultural backgrounds. During this translation work, there was a suggestion to use 'purify' instead. The translator puts importance on what Masahiro Oki means with the word, which is: Yoga teaches to find God within the self and make step-by-step efforts in practical daily-life aspects of body, mind, lifestyle and so on, in order to become able to interpret and treat everything as sacred. Along this line, the word 'sanctified' is used.

A dog will only recognise water as water. The *busshō* is the reverent *mind-heart that interprets water as a blessing from heaven and earth, the love of God.

Only with this reverent *mind-heart can the right way of thinking and acting arise, as well as the right way of resolving problems. In this sanctified *mind-heart, Heaven is born.

Prasāda (*hōetsu*) — the tenth stage

When we come to know the truth, feel gratitude and attain a mind of reverence, true joy can arise. Because yoga aims for this state, I call it 'happiness training'. As its distinctive feature, yoga teaches that God is within the self and that seeing this God is enlightenment. I believe that, when we are enlightened and see God within ourselves and others, we will be able to experience true joy (*hōetsu*).

My explanation may sound very difficult, but this is the true teaching of yoga. The goal, *hōetsu*, will be hard to attain. However, if you make the effort to correctly practise whatever stage it is, your body and mind will receive benefits accordingly. So, please try.